# Contents

$$\blacklozenge$$

# Introduction

✦

Protein is more than just fuel for muscles—it's the nutrient that keeps your body satisfied, energized, and strong. When you eat protein, your body takes longer to digest it compared to carbs or fat. That slower digestion helps you feel fuller for longer, which naturally reduces cravings and mindless snacking. This makes high-protein meals a powerful tool for anyone trying to manage weight.

Protein also protects your lean muscle. When you cut calories without enough protein, your body may break down muscle tissue for energy. Over time, that lowers your metabolism and makes it harder to keep weight off. A steady supply of protein ensures you burn fat while holding onto muscle, which keeps your metabolism active.

There's also a simple energy advantage. Your body uses more calories to digest protein than it does to process carbs or fat—a phenomenon known as the thermic effect of food. Even at rest, eating protein boosts how many calories you burn each day.

Finally, protein is the raw material your body needs to repair tissues, build enzymes, and support a strong immune system. Whether your goal is muscle gain, weight loss, or healthy aging, a protein-rich diet lays the foundation.

The promise of this cookbook is simple: when you build meals around protein, you make every calorie work harder for you. With recipes that balance flavor, convenience, and complete nutrition, you'll see why high protein isn't just a diet trend—it's a sustainable way to eat for life.

# The Problem

Most diets fail because they focus on restriction instead of nourishment. They cut calories or entire food groups, leaving you hungry, low on energy, and constantly fighting cravings. At the center of this problem is one key mistake: not enough protein. When protein is too low, your body doesn't feel satisfied, your muscles aren't protected, and your metabolism slows. This creates the perfect storm for yo-yo dieting—losing weight quickly, then regaining it just as fast.

Another issue is the lack of a clear prep strategy. Diet plans often hand you recipes without thinking about real life. You might be expected to cook three different meals a day, every day, with no plan for how to save time or stretch ingredients. That's unrealistic in a busy world. Without guidance on batch cooking, storage, and easy reheating, most people burn out before they ever see results.

Finally, many diets ignore flexibility. They don't offer substitutions for allergies or budgets, and they rarely show you how to adapt recipes to fit your personal protein needs. When your food doesn't match your lifestyle, it's easy to quit.

The truth is, lasting results require both the proper nutrients and a plan to make them practical. A high-protein diet gives your body what it needs, and a meal-prep approach makes it sustainable. This cookbook was designed to solve both problems—so you can stop cycling through diets that don't work and finally build a way of eating that does.

# The Fix

This cookbook was created to solve the two problems most diets overlook: insufficient protein and no realistic plan. Inside, you'll find more than 150 recipes—more than most other books in this category—so you'll never run out of ideas. Every recipe includes a complete nutrition label with protein, carbs, fats, fiber, calories, serving size in both US and metric, and even cost per serving. You'll know exactly what you're eating and how it fits into your goals.

To make eating high protein sustainable, this book is built around meal prep. Each recipe comes with clear storage and reheating instructions, plus icons that highlight batch-friendly, freezer-safe, one-pan, and budget meals. Weekly meal-prep maps and a 30-day plan are included so you can cook once and eat well all week without guesswork.

We've also added flexibility that other books leave out. A substitution matrix gives you options for gluten-free, dairy-free, nut-free, or vegan swaps. Dedicated chapters cover plant-powered protein, high-protein meals for active aging, and protein-dense, small-volume dishes that work for readers using GLP-1 medications. These tracks ensure the book meets you where you are, no matter your lifestyle or dietary needs.

This is more than a collection of recipes—it's a complete system to help you eat high protein in a way that's practical, affordable, and sustainable. With the right balance of nutrition, prep guidance, and flexibility, you finally have a resource that takes the guesswork out of eating for your health and goals.

# Quick Start

# How to Use the Book

✦

This book is designed to be simple from the very first page. Start with the protein calculator in Chapter 2. Use it to find your daily target based on your weight, activity level, and goals. Once you know your number, you can choose recipes that deliver the right amount of protein per meal. Each recipe clearly shows grams of protein per serving so you can hit your target without guesswork.

Next, get familiar with the icons used throughout the book. You'll see markers for one-pan, freezer-friendly, under-30-minutes, budget-friendly, and plant-based meals. These quick visual cues help you pick recipes that fit your time, tools, and lifestyle.

If you want a ready-made plan, head to the 30-day meal plan in Part IV. It combines recipes into balanced weeks with shopping lists and prep tips. For even more flexibility, use the weekly meal-prep maps. These show you how to cook a base recipe once and turn it into several different meals.

Finally, pay attention to the storage and reheating notes on each recipe. They'll guide you on how long a dish lasts in the fridge, how to freeze it safely, and the best way to bring it back to life.

Whether you follow the full plan or pick and choose recipes, the structure is here to make high-protein eating effortless. Use the tools, trust the process, and let the system work for you—so you spend less time worrying about food and more time enjoying it.

---

# Part

# I

# **Foundations**

---

# Chapter 1

# The Importance of Protein

$\blacklozenge$

Protein is the foundation of every cell in your body. It builds and repairs muscle, supports your immune system, and provides the building blocks for hormones and enzymes. But beyond these biological roles, protein has powerful effects on how you feel day to day and how your body manages weight.

One of the most important benefits is satiety. Protein takes longer to break down than carbohydrates or fat, so it keeps you fuller for longer. This means fewer energy crashes and less mindless snacking between meals. For people trying to manage their weight, that sense of fullness can be the difference between sticking to a plan and giving up.

Protein also protects muscle during weight loss. When calories are reduced without enough protein, the body burns not only fat but also lean tissue. Losing muscle slows your metabolism and makes it harder to maintain results. A protein-rich diet helps preserve muscle mass, keeping your metabolism steady while you lose fat.

As you age, protein becomes even more critical. Natural muscle loss can lead to weakness, falls, and slower recovery from illness or injury. A higher protein intake supports strength, balance, and independence well into later years.

Finally, protein has a thermic advantage: your body uses more energy to digest protein than it does for carbs or fats. This small but steady boost adds up over time, making it easier to maintain a healthy weight.

In short, protein isn't just about building muscle—it's about fueling a healthier, stronger, and more resilient body for life.

# Protein vs. Other Macronutrients on Satiety

Not all calories affect hunger the same way. Studies consistently show that protein provides the strongest satiety signal compared to carbohydrates and fat. When you eat a high-protein meal, your body releases hormones like peptide YY and GLP-1 that help you feel full and satisfied. Carbohydrates can give quick energy, but they also trigger sharp rises and falls in blood sugar that leave you hungry again within a few hours. Fat contributes to flavor and slows digestion slightly, but it lacks the appetite-regulating impact of protein. This is why a meal centered around lean protein keeps cravings at bay far longer than a carb-heavy snack or a high-fat treat.

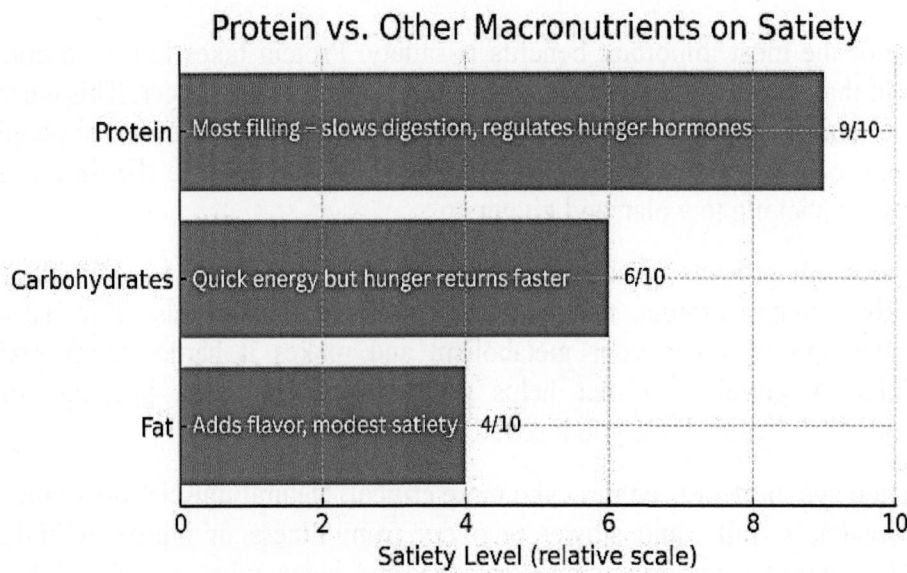

*Descriptive text: Horizontal bar chart*

- *X-axis: Level of satiety (short, moderate, long).*

- *Y-axis: Macronutrients (Protein, Carbohydrates, Fat).*

- *Bars:*

   - *Protein: Longest bar, labeled "Most filling – slows digestion, regulates hunger hormones."*

- *Carbohydrates: Medium bar, labeled "Quick energy but hunger returns faster."*

- *Fat: Shorter bar, labeled "Adds flavor, modest satiety."*

# Protein & Metabolism Boost

Protein also has a unique advantage called the thermic effect of food. Your body must work to digest and process every calorie you eat, but the effort required varies by macronutrient. Protein has the highest thermic effect—roughly 20–30% of its calories are burned just in the process of digestion. In comparison, carbs use about 5–10% and fats only 0–3%. This means that 100 calories from protein results in a smaller net calorie impact than 100 calories from carbs or fat. Over time, consistently eating protein-rich meals supports a slightly higher daily calorie burn, even at rest.

Together, the satiety effect and thermic advantage explain why high-protein diets are linked to easier weight control, better appetite management, and stronger long-term results. Protein works harder for your body than any other nutrient.

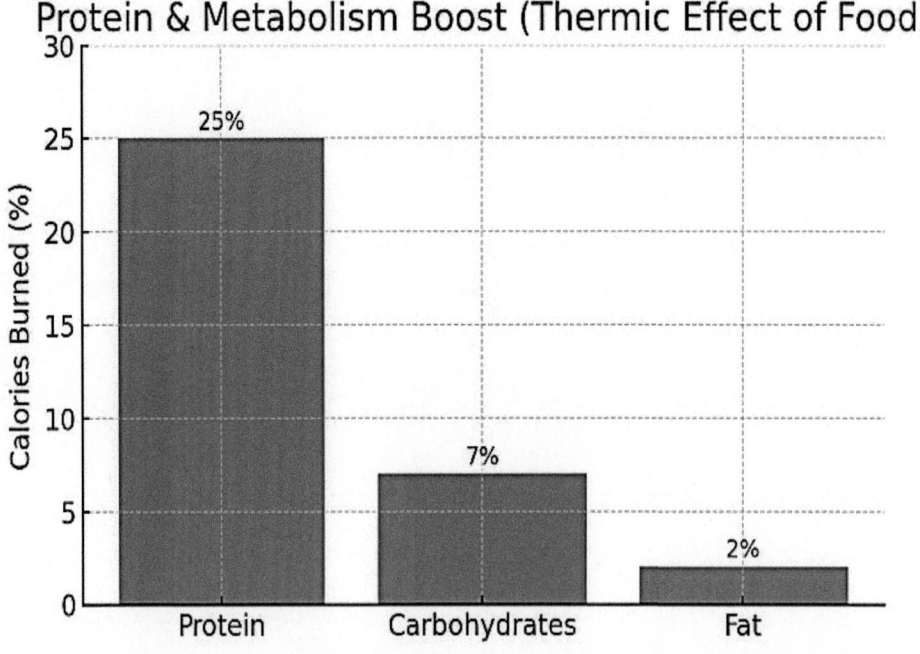

**Protein & Metabolism Boost (Thermic Effect of Food)**

**\*Protein burns the most energy during digestion, giving your metabolism a steady lift.**

*Descriptive Text: Simple bar graph with calories burned during digestion per 100 calories eaten.*

- *X-axis: Macronutrient type.*

- *Y-axis: Percentage of calories burned through digestion (thermic effect).*

- *Bars:*

  - *Protein: 20–30% (highlighted in a bold shade).*

  - *Carbohydrates: 5–10%.*

  - *Fat: 0–3%.*

# Mini Science Call-Outs

## Protein and Satiety

Research shows that protein-rich meals increase the release of appetite-regulating hormones like peptide YY and GLP-1, which help you feel full and satisfied. In contrast, carbohydrate-heavy meals can trigger sharp blood sugar spikes and crashes that leave you hungry again soon after eating (Weigle et al., 2005).

## Protein and Weight Control

A high-protein diet supports weight management by reducing daily calorie intake without intentional restriction. Studies demonstrate that raising protein intake to around 25–30% of calories can naturally reduce hunger and lead to greater fat loss while preserving lean body mass (Westerterp-Plantenga et al., 2009).

## Protein and Muscle Preservation

When people lose weight, they risk losing muscle along with fat. Adequate protein intake helps preserve lean mass, keeping metabolism steady and improving long-term weight maintenance (Paddon-Jones et al., 2008).

## Protein and Healthy Aging

Older adults need more protein to counteract age-related muscle loss, known as sarcopenia. Diets with higher protein levels improve strength, mobility, and independence in older populations (Bauer et al., 2013).

## Protein and Energy Expenditure

Protein has the highest thermic effect of all macronutrients. Roughly 20–30% of protein calories are burned during digestion, compared to 5–10% for carbohydrates and 0–3% for fats. This "metabolic boost" supports energy balance and makes protein especially efficient for weight control (Halton & Hu, 2004).

Together, these findings show that protein is not just about muscle building—it's a central nutrient for satiety, weight management, and long-term health.

# Chapter 2

# Find Your Protein Target

✦

## Protein Target Calculator

The simplest way to set your protein goal is to calculate it based on body weight and overall goal. Protein needs are best expressed in grams per pound (or kilogram) of body weight. This approach gives you a target that adapts to your size and activity rather than a one-size-fits-all rule.

## Step 1: Weigh yourself.

Use your current body weight in pounds (or kilograms).

## Step 2: Choose your goal.

- **Fat Loss:** Aim for 0.8–1.0 grams of protein per pound (1.8–2.2 g/kg). A higher intake helps preserve muscle while reducing calories.

- **Maintenance/General Health:** Aim for 0.6–0.8 grams per pound (1.4–1.8 g/kg). This range supports steady energy, satiety, and long-term health.

- **Muscle Gain/Recomposition:** Aim for 1.0–1.2 grams per pound (2.2–2.6 g/kg). Extra protein provides building blocks for new muscle while supporting recovery.

## Step 3: Do the math.

Multiply your body weight by the recommended number for your goal.

- *Example*: 170 lb × 0.8 = 136 g protein/day (fat loss target).

- *Example:* 65 kg × 2.0 = 130 g protein/day (fat loss target).

# Step 4: Divide by meals.

Spread your protein across 3–5 meals. For the 170 lb example, 136 g ÷ 4 meals = about 34 g protein per meal.

With this calculator, you can quickly identify your daily target and use the recipe macros in this book to build meals that consistently hit it.

## Find Your Protein Target

Step 1: Write your body weight: _____ lb   or   _____ kg

Step 2: Choose your goal:

• Fat Loss: 0.8–1.0 g per lb    (1.8–2.2 g per kg)

• Maintenance: 0.6–0.8 g per lb    (1.4–1.8 g per kg)

• Muscle Gain: 1.0–1.2 g per lb    (2.2–2.6 g per kg)

Step 3: Multiply weight × protein factor = _____ g protein/day

Step 4: Divide by meals: _____ ÷ _____ meals = _____ g protein/meal

# Example Daily Menus

It can be difficult to picture what different protein targets look like in real meals. Here are three sample menus that show how you might spread protein across the day depending on your needs.

## 20 g Protein per Meal (≈80 g/day)

- **Breakfast:** Greek yogurt with berries and chia seeds.
- **Lunch:** Turkey and avocado wrap with whole-grain tortilla.
- **Snack:** Cottage cheese with sliced cucumber.
- **Dinner:** Grilled salmon with quinoa and roasted vegetables.

## 30 g Protein per Meal (≈120 g/day)

- **Breakfast:** Protein smoothie with whey powder, almond butter, and banana.
- **Lunch:** Chicken burrito bowl with brown rice and black beans.
- **Snack:** Hummus with edamame and whole-grain crackers.
- **Dinner:** Lean beef chili with kidney beans and mixed greens.

## 40 g Protein per Meal (≈160 g/day)

- **Breakfast:** Omelet with four eggs, spinach, and feta plus turkey sausage.
- **Lunch:** Grilled chicken breast, lentil salad, and roasted sweet potatoes.
- **Snack:** Protein shake with Greek yogurt and peanut butter.
- **Dinner:** Baked cod with quinoa pilaf, steamed broccoli, and a chickpea side salad.

These menus are not strict meal plans but simple examples. Use them to visualize how much food it takes to reach different protein goals. With recipes in this book, you'll be able to build your own days in the same way—balancing meals so that hitting your protein target becomes automatic.

# Sidebar: How to Adjust as You Age, Train, or Recover from Illness

Protein needs aren't static—they shift with age, activity, and health. Understanding when to adjust helps you stay on track long term.

## As You Age

Starting around age 40, the body gradually loses muscle, a process called sarcopenia. To counter this, older adults benefit from the higher end of protein ranges, about 0.8–1.0 g per pound (1.8–2.2 g/kg). Spreading protein evenly across meals supports muscle retention and bone health.

## When Training Hard

If you lift weights, run long distances, or train for endurance events, your muscles need more raw material for repair and growth. Athletes and active individuals do best at 1.0–1.2 g per pound (2.2–2.6 g/kg). Consistency matters—fueling every meal with a strong protein source helps recovery and performance.

## During Illness or Recovery

Injury, surgery, or illness can increase protein needs as the body works to heal. Protein provides the building blocks for tissue repair and helps preserve strength during periods of reduced activity. In these times, aim for the higher end of your recommended range and divide intake across 4–5 smaller meals to improve absorption.

Adjusting your protein target to match life's stages ensures your diet always supports your body's changing demands. Rather than seeing protein as fixed, treat it as a flexible tool you can dial up or down depending on your goals and circumstances.

# Chapter 3

# Your High-Protein Kitchen

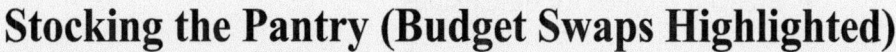

## Stocking the Pantry (Budget Swaps Highlighted)

A well-stocked kitchen makes high-protein eating easier and less expensive. Keeping a mix of fresh, frozen, and shelf-stable protein sources on hand means you can always throw together a balanced meal without last-minute stress.

## Proteins to Keep in Stock

- **Canned tuna, salmon, and chicken:** Affordable, long-lasting, and ready in minutes. *Budget swap: choose store brands packed in water instead of specialty varieties.*

- **Eggs and liquid egg whites:** Versatile, inexpensive, and protein-packed. *Budget swap: buy bulk cartons of egg whites if you use them often.*

- **Greek yogurt and cottage cheese:** Great for snacks or recipe bases. *Budget swap: buy large tubs rather than single-serve cups.*

- **Dry or canned beans and lentils:** Plant-based protein staples. *Budget swap: cook large batches of dried beans for pennies on the dollar.*

- **Frozen chicken breast, turkey, or fish fillets:** Convenient and often cheaper than fresh cuts. *Budget swap: family-size bags save more per pound.*

- **Protein powders:** Useful for shakes or baking. *Budget swap:*

*unflavored or single-ingredient powders are usually cheaper than flavored blends.*

## Supporting Staples

- Whole grains like oats, brown rice, and quinoa.

- Healthy fats such as olive oil, peanut butter, and nuts. *Budget swap: buy store-brand nut butters or bulk packs of nuts.*

- Freezer veggies for quick sides.

Stocking these basics keeps meal prep flexible. With protein-rich building blocks and budget-friendly swaps, you'll be ready to make recipes from this book anytime without breaking the bank.

# Substitution Matrix: Dairy-Free, Gluten-Free, Nut-Free, Vegan Swaps

High-protein eating should be flexible enough to fit any lifestyle or dietary need. Use this substitution matrix to adapt recipes without losing nutrition or flavor.

## Dairy-Free

- **Greek yogurt** → coconut yogurt (add a scoop of protein powder to match protein content).
- **Cottage cheese** → silken tofu blended with lemon juice for creaminess.
- **Milk** → fortified soy milk (highest protein of plant milks).
- **Cheese** → dairy-free cheese plus nutritional yeast for flavor.

## Gluten-Free

- **Wheat tortillas** → corn tortillas or gluten-free wraps.
- **Pasta** → chickpea or lentil pasta (higher protein than wheat).
- **Breadcrumbs** → crushed rice cakes or gluten-free oats pulsed in a blender.
- **Soy sauce** → tamari or coconut aminos.

## Nut-Free

- **Almond butter** → sunflower seed or pumpkin seed butter.
- **Chopped nuts in recipes** → roasted chickpeas or toasted seeds.
- **Nut milks** → oat milk or soy milk for creaminess.
- **Nut-based protein bars** → seed-based bars or homemade oat + seed options.

# Vegan

- **Chicken breast** → extra-firm tofu, tempeh, or seitan.

- **Ground beef/turkey** → lentils, crumbled tempeh, or textured vegetable protein.

- **Eggs in baking** → flax or chia "egg" (1 tbsp seed + 3 tbsp water).

- **Whey protein** → pea, hemp, or rice protein powder.

With these swaps, every recipe in this book can be tailored to fit your dietary preferences—without sacrificing protein or convenience.

# Tools & Appliances (Air Fryer, Slow Cooker, Instant Pot, Sheet-Pan)

The right tools make meal prep faster, easier, and more enjoyable. While you don't need a kitchen full of gadgets, a few key appliances can save hours and open up more recipe options.

## Air Fryer

Cooks food quickly with minimal oil, delivering crisp textures similar to frying. Great for chicken, fish, vegetables, and even high-protein snacks like chickpeas or tofu bites.

## Slow Cooker

It's perfect for set-it-and-forget-it meals. It works best with soups, stews, and big-batch proteins like shredded chicken or pulled turkey. It's also ideal for prepping several days' worth of meals at once.

## Instant Pot (or any pressure cooker)

It dramatically cuts cooking time. You can make tender meats, beans, and grains in a fraction of the time compared to the stovetop. It also functions as a slow cooker, steamer, and rice cooker, making it one of the most versatile kitchen tools.

## Sheet-Pan

A simple sheet pan can transform weeknight cooking. By roasting protein, vegetables, and grains together, you get balanced meals with minimal cleanup. This pan is perfect for one-pan recipes and batch cooking.

Even if you only have basic pots, pans, and a skillet, you can make every recipe in this book. These tools simply give you more flexibility to choose the cooking style that fits your schedule and prep style.

# Prep Basics: Containers, Freezing, Labeling

Meal prep only works if your food stays fresh, organized, and easy to grab. Investing a little time in storage basics makes the whole system smoother.

## Containers

Choose a mix of portion-sized and family-sized containers. Glass containers with snap lids are ideal because they don't stain, seal tightly, and reheat well. BPA-free plastic is lighter and budget-friendly. Divided containers are useful for keeping protein and sides separate.

## Freezing

Not every recipe freezes well, but many proteins, soups, and casseroles do. Always cool food completely before freezing to prevent ice crystals. Freeze in single portions when possible so you can thaw only what you need. Use freezer bags for flat storage—label and stack them like files to save space.

## Labeling

Always date your containers before refrigerating or freezing. A simple piece of masking tape and a marker works fine. Note the dish name, prep date, and "use by" date (generally 3–4 days in the fridge, up to 3 months in the freezer). Clear labeling prevents mystery meals and wasted food.

With the right containers, smart freezing habits, and clear labeling, you'll build a system that keeps meals safe, flavorful, and ready when you are. These small details transform meal prep from a chore into a sustainable routine.

# Part
# II
# Recipes

# Chapter 4

# Breakfasts & On-the-Go

———————————— ✦ ————————————

Mornings set the tone for the entire day, and starting with a protein-rich breakfast helps you feel energized, satisfied, and ready to focus. This chapter brings you more than 25 recipes designed to fit real-life mornings—whether you have five minutes before running out the door or a little extra time on the weekend.

You'll find:

- **Quick grab-and-go options** like parfaits, smoothies, and muffins that can be prepped in advance.

- **Hearty make-ahead meals** such as frittatas, egg bakes, and breakfast burritos that reheat beautifully for busy mornings.

- **Balanced sweet and savory choices** so you can enjoy variety without sacrificing nutrition.

- **On-the-go snacks** like protein bars, energy bites, and portable wraps to keep hunger in check between meals.

Every recipe includes full macros, meal-prep tips, and storage guidance. Plant-based, gluten-free, and dairy-free swaps are highlighted so you can easily adapt to your needs. With these options, breakfast becomes more than a rushed routine—it's a dependable way to reach your protein goals from the very first meal of the day.

# Recipe Icons Guide

🔍 **One-Pan**
Cook the whole meal in a single pan —
less cleanup, more convenience.

❄️ **Freezer-Friendly**
Can be stored in the freezer for later;
reheats well.

💲 **Budget-Friendly**
Costs under $4 per serving with
common ingredients.

⏱️ **Under 30 Minutes**
From prep to plate in half an hour or
less.

⭐ **30+ g Protein**
Each serving delivers at least 30 grams
of protein.

🌱 **Plant-Based**
Fully vegetarian or vegan protein
sources.

# Almond Butter Protein Smoothie Bowl

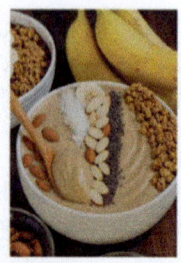

Servings: 1  |  Prep Time: 10 min  |  Total Time: 10 min
Icons: ⏱ Under 30 Min   🌱 Plant-Based (with swaps)

## Ingredients

- 1 frozen banana
- 1 scoop vanilla protein powder
- 1 cup unsweetened almond milk
- 2 tbsp almond butter
- ¼ cup granola
- 2 tbsp sliced almonds
- 1 tbsp chia seeds

## Directions

1. Blend banana, protein powder, almond milk, and almond butter until thick and smooth.
2. Pour into a bowl; top with granola, almonds, and chia seeds.

### Nutrition (per serving)

- Calories: 400
- Protein: 30 g
- Carbs: 35 g (Fiber: 8 g)
- Fat: 16 g

### Substitutions

- Nut-free: use sunflower butter and pumpkin seeds.

### Storage & Prep

- Best enjoyed fresh.
- Prep toppings in advance for faster mornings.

# Greek Yogurt Protein Parfait

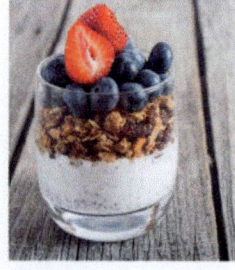

Servings: 1  |  Prep Time: 5 min  |  Total Time: 5 min
Icons: 🌱 Plant-Based (with swaps)  ⏱ Under 30 Min   $ Budget-Friendly

## Ingredients

- 1 cup plain nonfat Greek yogurt
- ½ cup mixed berries (fresh or frozen)
- 2 tbsp granola
- 1 tbsp chia seeds
- 1 scoop vanilla whey or plant protein powder
- 1 tsp honey or maple syrup (optional)

## Directions

1. In a bowl or jar, mix Greek yogurt with protein powder until smooth.
2. Layer yogurt, berries, and granola.
3. Sprinkle chia seeds on top and drizzle with honey if desired.

### Nutrition (per serving)

- Calories: 310
- Protein: 34 g
- Carbs: 32 g (Fiber: 8 g)
- Fat: 7 g

### Substitutions

- Dairy-free: use coconut yogurt + plant protein.
- Nut-free: choose nut-free granola.

### Storage & Prep

- Assemble in mason jars for grab-and-go breakfasts.
- Keeps up to 2 days in the fridge.

# Veggie Egg Muffins

Servings: 6 muffins (3 servings)  |  Prep Time: 10 min  |  Cook Time: 20 min  |  Total Time: 30 min
Icons: 🔍 One-Pan  ⏱ Under 30 Min  ❄ Freezer-Friendly  $ Budget-Friendly

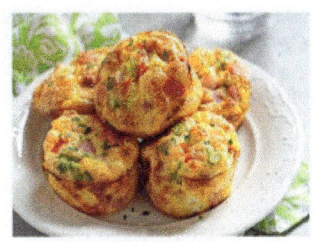

## Ingredients

- 6 large eggs
- ¼ cup low-fat milk (or unsweetened soy milk)
- ½ cup diced bell peppers
- ½ cup chopped spinach
- ¼ cup diced onion
- ½ cup shredded low-fat cheddar cheese
- Salt & pepper, to taste
- Cooking spray or olive oil for greasing

**Nutrition (per serving = 2 muffins)**

- Calories: 190
- Protein: 20 g
- Carbs: 4 g (Fiber: 1 g)
- Fat: 10 g

## Directions

1. Preheat oven to 350°F (175°C). Lightly grease a 6-cup muffin tin.
2. In a bowl, whisk eggs and milk until smooth.
3. Stir in bell peppers, spinach, onion, cheese, salt, and pepper.
4. Divide mixture evenly into muffin cups.
5. Bake 18–20 minutes, until eggs are set and tops are lightly golden.
6. Cool slightly before removing from tin.

**Substitutions**

- Dairy-free: swap soy milk + dairy-free cheese.
- Plant-based: use chickpea flour batter (1 cup chickpea flour + 1 cup water) instead of eggs.

**Storage & Prep**

- Refrigerate up to 4 days in an airtight container.
- Freeze up to 2 months; reheat in microwave for 60–90 seconds.

# Chocolate Peanut Butter Protein Smoothie

Servings: 1  |  Prep Time: 5 min  |  Total Time: 5 min
Icons: ⏱ Under 30 Min  🌱 Plant-Based (with swaps)  $ Budget-Friendly

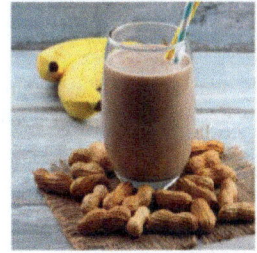

## Ingredients

- 1 cup unsweetened almond milk (or dairy milk)
- 1 frozen banana
- 1 scoop chocolate protein powder (whey or plant-based)
- 2 tbsp peanut butter
- 1 tbsp cocoa powder
- ½ cup ice cubes

**Nutrition (per serving)**

- Calories: 370
- Protein: 32 g
- Carbs: 32 g (Fiber: 6 g)
- Fat: 14 g

## Directions

1. Combine all ingredients in a blender.
2. Blend until smooth and creamy.
3. Pour into a glass and enjoy immediately.

**Substitutions**

- Nut-free: use sunflower seed butter.
- Lower-calorie: reduce to 1 tbsp peanut butter.

**Storage & Prep**

- Best consumed fresh.
- Freeze banana in advance for creaminess.

# Turkey Sausage Breakfast Burritos

Servings: 4 | Prep Time: 15 min | Cook Time: 15 min | Total Time: 30 min
Icons: 🔍 One-Pan ❄ Freezer-Friendly $ Budget-Friendly

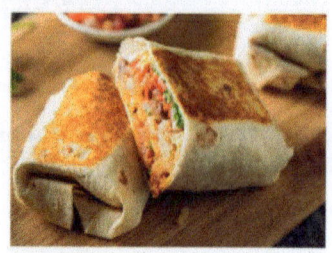

### Ingredients

- 8 oz lean ground turkey sausage
- 6 large eggs
- ¼ cup low-fat milk
- ½ cup shredded cheddar cheese
- ½ cup diced bell peppers
- ½ cup diced onion
- 4 large whole-wheat tortillas

### Directions

1. In a skillet, cook turkey sausage until browned.
2. Add peppers and onion; sauté until softened.
3. In a bowl, whisk eggs with milk, then pour into skillet. Scramble until set.
4. Stir in cheese.
5. Divide filling among tortillas and roll into burritos.

### Nutrition (per burrito)

- Calories: 390
- Protein: 33 g
- Carbs: 29 g (Fiber: 6 g)
- Fat: 15 g

### Substitutions

- Dairy-free: use plant milk and dairy-free cheese.
- Gluten-free: use gluten-free tortillas.

### Storage & Prep

- Wrap tightly in foil, refrigerate up to 4 days.
- Freeze up to 2 months; reheat in microwave or oven.

# Cottage Cheese Pancakes

Servings: 2 | Prep Time: 10 min | Cook Time: 10 min | Total Time: 20 min
Icons: ⏱ Under 30 Min $ Budget-Friendly

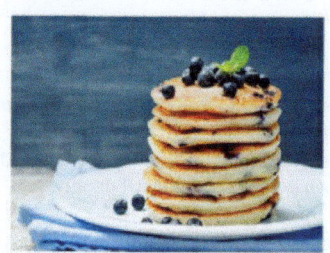

### Ingredients

- 1 cup low-fat cottage cheese
- 2 large eggs
- ½ cup rolled oats
- 1 tsp vanilla extract
- 1 tsp baking powder
- Cooking spray or butter for pan

### Directions

1. Blend cottage cheese, eggs, oats, vanilla, and baking powder until smooth.
2. Heat a skillet, spray lightly, and pour small pancakes.
3. Cook 2–3 minutes per side until golden.
4. Serve with berries or sugar-free syrup.

### Nutrition (per serving)

- Calories: 290
- Protein: 28 g
- Carbs: 28 g (Fiber: 4 g)
- Fat: 7 g

### Substitutions

- Gluten-free oats for GF option.
- Dairy-free cottage cheese substitute for vegan option (lower protein).

### Storage & Prep

- Refrigerate up to 3 days.
- Freeze cooked pancakes, reheat in toaster.

# Smoked Salmon & Egg Wrap

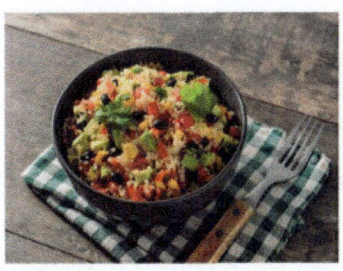

Servings: 1 | Prep Time: 5 min | Total Time: 5 min
Icons: ⏱ Under 30 Min  $ Budget-Friendly

## Ingredients

- 1 whole-wheat tortilla
- 2 hard-boiled eggs, sliced
- 2 oz smoked salmon
- 1 tbsp light cream cheese
- ¼ cup spinach leaves

## Directions

1. Spread cream cheese on tortilla.
2. Layer spinach, salmon, and egg slices.
3. Roll into a wrap and slice in half.

## Nutrition (per serving)

- Calories: 330
- Protein: 29 g
- Carbs: 26 g (Fiber: 5 g)
- Fat: 12 g

## Substitutions

- Dairy-free: use dairy-free cream cheese.
- Gluten-free: swap GF tortilla.

## Storage & Prep

- Best eaten fresh; store up to 24 hours wrapped tightly.

# Savory Quinoa Breakfast Bowl

Servings: 2 | Prep Time: 10 min | Cook Time: 20 min | Total Time: 30 min
Icons: ⌕ One-Pan  ⏱ Under 30 Min  🌱 Plant-Based (with swaps)

## Ingredients

- 1 cup cooked quinoa
- 2 fried or poached eggs
- ½ cup black beans
- ½ avocado, sliced
- ½ cup sautéed spinach
- Salsa or hot sauce, to taste

## Directions

1. Divide quinoa into bowls.
2. Top with beans, spinach, and eggs.
3. Add avocado slices and drizzle with salsa.

## Nutrition (per serving)

- Calories: 370
- Protein: 24 g
- Carbs: 40 g (Fiber: 9 g)
- Fat: 14 g

## Substitutions

- Vegan: swap eggs for tofu scramble.
- Budget: use canned beans and bulk quinoa.

## Storage & Prep

- Prep quinoa and beans in advance.
- Assemble fresh or reheat base and top with eggs.

# High-Protein Banana Muffins

Servings: 12 muffins (6 servings)  |  Prep Time: 10 min  |  Cook Time: 20 min  | Total Time: 30 min

Icons: ❄ Freezer-Friendly  $ Budget-Friendly

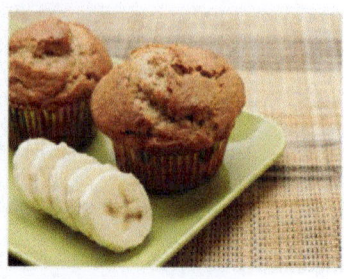

## Ingredients

- 2 ripe bananas, mashed
- 2 large eggs
- 1 cup rolled oats, blended into flour
- 1 scoop vanilla protein powder
- 1 tsp baking powder
- ½ tsp cinnamon
- 2 tbsp honey or maple syrup

## Nutrition (per serving = 2 muffins)

- Calories: 210
- Protein: 20 g
- Carbs: 27 g (Fiber: 4 g)
- Fat: 5 g

## Directions

1. Preheat oven to 350°F (175°C). Line a muffin tin.
2. Mix bananas, eggs, oats, protein powder, baking powder, cinnamon, and honey until smooth.
3. Divide batter into 12 muffin cups.
4. Bake 18–20 minutes until firm.

## Substitutions

- Dairy-free protein powder if needed.
- Gluten-free oats for GF option.

## Storage & Prep

- Refrigerate up to 5 days.
- Freeze up to 2 months.

# Cottage Cheese Berry Bowl

Servings: 1  |  Prep Time: 5 min  |  Total Time: 5 min

Icons: ⏱ Under 30 Min  $ Budget-Friendly

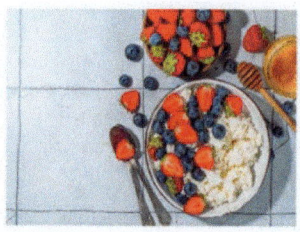

## Ingredients
- 1 cup low-fat cottage cheese
- ½ cup strawberries, sliced
- ½ cup blueberries
- 1 tbsp ground flaxseed
- 1 tsp honey (optional)

## Nutrition (per serving)

- Calories: 260
- Protein: 28 g
- Carbs: 20 g (Fiber: 5 g)
- Fat: 7 g

## Directions
1. Place cottage cheese in a bowl.
2. Top with berries and flaxseed.
3. Drizzle with honey if desired.

## Substitutions

- Dairy-free: swap for soy-based yogurt + protein powder.

## Storage & Prep

- Best fresh, but can be prepped in advance and refrigerated up to 2 days.

# Savory Cottage Cheese Protein Waffles

Servings: 4 waffles (2 servings)  |  Prep Time: 10 min  |  Cook Time: 10 min  |  Total Time: 20 min
Icons: ⏱ Under 30 Min  🔍 One-Pan  $ Budget-Friendly

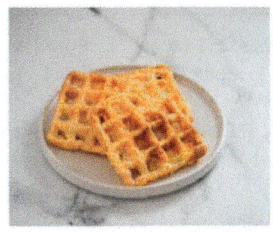

## Ingredients

- 1 cup low-fat cottage cheese
- 2 large eggs
- ½ cup rolled oats
- 1 scoop unflavored or savory protein powder
- ½ tsp baking powder
- ¼ tsp garlic powder
- ¼ tsp salt
- Cooking spray for waffle iron

**Nutrition (per serving = 2 waffles)**

- Calories: 290
- Protein: 32 g
- Carbs: 22 g (Fiber: 3 g)
- Fat: 8 g

## Directions

1. Blend cottage cheese, eggs, oats, protein powder, baking powder, garlic powder, and salt until smooth.
2. Heat and lightly grease a waffle iron.
3. Pour in batter and cook 3–5 minutes until golden brown.
4. Serve plain, or top with avocado and smoked salmon for extra protein.

**Substitutions**

- Dairy-free: use silken tofu instead of cottage cheese and plant protein powder.
- Gluten-free: swap oats for certified GF oats.

**Storage & Prep**

- Refrigerate up to 4 days; reheat in toaster.
- Freeze up to 2 months; toast directly from frozen.

# High-Protein Breakfast Quesadilla

Servings: 2  |  Prep Time: 10 min  |  Cook Time: 10 min  |  Total Time: 20 min
Icons: 🔍 One-Pan  ⏱ Under 30 Min  ❄ Freezer-Friendly  $ Budget-Friendly

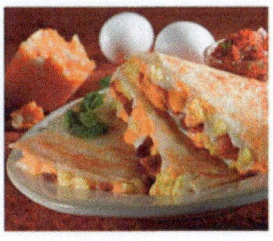

## Ingredients

- 4 large whole-wheat tortillas
- 4 large eggs
- ½ cup egg whites
- ½ cup shredded cheddar cheese (or dairy-free alternative)
- ½ cup black beans, rinsed and drained
- ½ cup diced bell peppers
- 1 tbsp olive oil or cooking spray

**Nutrition (per serving)**

- Calories: 360
- Protein: 32 g
- Carbs: 32 g (Fiber: 8 g)
- Fat: 12 g

## Directions

1. Heat skillet over medium and lightly oil.
2. Whisk eggs and egg whites together, then scramble until just set.
3. Place a tortilla in skillet, sprinkle with cheese, eggs, beans, and peppers, then top with a second tortilla.
4. Cook 2–3 minutes per side until golden and crisp.
5. Cut into wedges and serve warm.

**Substitutions**

- Gluten-free: use GF tortillas.
- Vegan: scramble crumbled tofu with spices instead of eggs.

**Storage & Prep**

- Refrigerate up to 3 days; reheat in skillet for crispness.
- Freeze individually wrapped wedges up to 2 months.

# Black Bean Breakfast Tacos

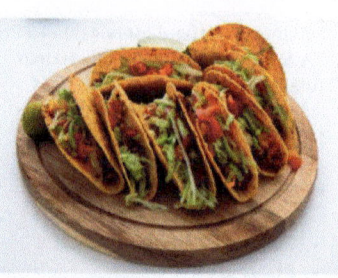

Servings: 2 (4 tacos)  |  Prep Time: 10 min  |  Cook Time: 10 min  |  Total Time: 20 min
Icons: 🌱 Plant-Based  🔍 One-Pan  $ Budget-Friendly

## Ingredients

- 1 cup black beans, rinsed and drained
- ½ tsp cumin
- ½ tsp chili powder
- ½ cup diced peppers
- 4 small corn tortillas
- ¼ cup salsa
- 2 tbsp crumbled queso fresco (optional)

## Directions

1. Heat skillet, sauté beans with spices and peppers 5–6 minutes.
2. Warm tortillas.
3. Fill with bean mixture, salsa, and cheese if using.

### Nutrition (per 2 tacos)

- Calories: 270
- Protein: 21 g
- Carbs: 36 g (Fiber: 9 g)
- Fat: 5 g

### Substitutions

- Vegan: skip cheese or use plant-based cheese.

### Storage & Prep

- Bean mixture refrigerates up to 4 days. Assemble tacos fresh.

# Protein-Packed Breakfast Cookies

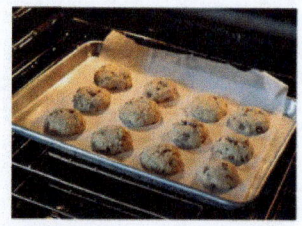

Servings: 12 cookies  |  Prep Time: 10 min  |  Cook Time: 15 min  |  Total Time: 25 min
Icons: ❄ Freezer-Friendly  🌱 Plant-Based  $ Budget-Friendly

## Ingredients

- 2 ripe bananas, mashed
- 1 cup rolled oats
- 1 scoop vanilla plant protein powder
- ¼ cup peanut butter
- ¼ cup raisins or cranberries
- 1 tsp cinnamon

## Directions

1. Preheat oven to 350°F (175°C). Line baking sheet with parchment.
2. Mix bananas, oats, protein powder, peanut butter, raisins, and cinnamon.
3. Scoop onto sheet, flatten slightly.
4. Bake 12–15 minutes until firm.

### Nutrition (per cookie)

- Calories: 120
- Protein: 7 g
- Carbs: 15 g (Fiber: 3 g)
- Fat: 4 g

### Substitutions

- Nut-free: use sunflower seed butter.

### Storage & Prep

- Refrigerate up to 1 week.
- Freeze up to 2 months.

# Greek Breakfast Bowl

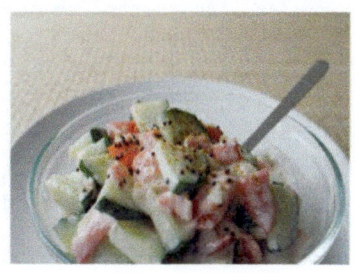

**Servings: 1 | Prep Time: 10 min | Total Time: 10 min**
**Icons:** ⏱ Under 30 Min   $ Budget-Friendly

## Ingredients

- 1 cup cooked quinoa
- ½ cup Greek yogurt
- ¼ cup chickpeas, rinsed
- ¼ cup diced cucumber
- ¼ cup cherry tomatoes, halved
- 1 tbsp olive oil
- Pinch of oregano and salt

**Nutrition (per serving)**

- Calories: 340
- Protein: 27 g
- Carbs: 35 g (Fiber: 7 g)
- Fat: 10 g

**Substitutions**

- Vegan: replace yogurt with plant-based yogur

## Directions

1. In a bowl, layer quinoa, Greek yogurt, chickpeas, cucumber, and tomatoes.
2. Drizzle with olive oil and sprinkle with oregano.

**Storage & Prep**

- Assemble fresh; keeps up to 2 days in fridge.

# Turkey & Egg Breakfast Skillet

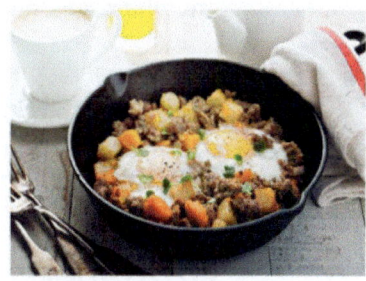

**Servings: 2 | Prep Time: 10 min | Cook Time: 15 min | Total Time: 25 min**
**Icons:** 🍳 One-Pan   ⏱ Under 30 Min   $ Budget-Friendly

## Ingredients

- 6 oz lean ground turkey
- ½ cup diced sweet potato
- ½ cup diced bell peppers
- ¼ cup onion, chopped
- 2 large eggs
- 1 tbsp olive oil

**Nutrition (per serving)**

- Calories: 330
- Protein: 29 g
- Carbs: 22 g (Fiber: 4 g)
- Fat: 14 g

**Substitutions**

- Plant-based: use tofu instead of turkey.

## Directions

1. Heat oil in skillet, cook turkey until browned.
2. Add sweet potato, peppers, and onion; cook until tender.
3. Make two wells, crack in eggs, cover and cook until eggs are set.

**Storage & Prep**

- Best fresh; can refrigerate leftovers up to 2 days.

# Chapter 5

# Lunches & Bowls

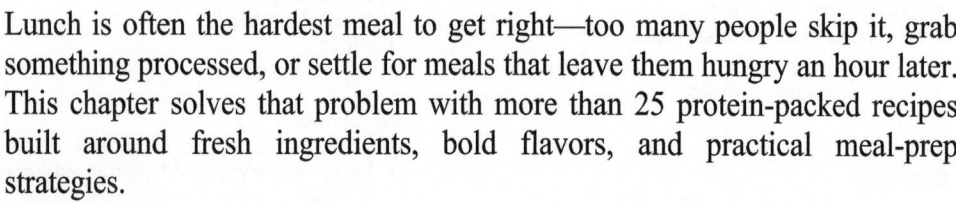

Lunch is often the hardest meal to get right—too many people skip it, grab something processed, or settle for meals that leave them hungry an hour later. This chapter solves that problem with more than 25 protein-packed recipes built around fresh ingredients, bold flavors, and practical meal-prep strategies.

You'll find:

- **Balanced bowls** that layer proteins, grains, and vegetables for lasting fullness.

- **Portable salads and wraps** that travel well to work, school, or anywhere you need fuel on the go.

- **Plant-based power meals** with lentils, tofu, and chickpeas designed to hit 25–30 grams of protein per serving.

- **Quick-prep options** that can be made in 30 minutes or less for busy days.

- **Freezer-friendly batch meals** that let you cook once and enjoy several days of effortless lunches.

Each recipe comes with full macros, budget-friendly swaps, and clear prep instructions so you can stay on track without stress. These lunches are designed not just to get you through the afternoon, but to keep you energized and satisfied until dinner.

# Recipe Icons Guide

🔍 **One-Pan**
Cook the whole meal in a single pan —
less cleanup, more convenience.

🕐 **Under 30 Minutes**
From prep to plate in half an hour or
less.

❄️ **Freezer-Friendly**
Can be stored in the freezer for later;
reheats well.

⭐ **30+ g Protein**
Each serving delivers at least 30 grams
of protein.

$ **Budget-Friendly**
Costs under $4 per serving with
common ingredients.

🌱 **Plant-Based**
Fully vegetarian or vegan protein
sources.

# High-Protein Chicken Burrito Bowls

Servings: 4  |  Prep Time: 15 min  |  Cook
Time: 20 min  |  Total Time: 35 min
Icons: 🔍 One-Pan  ❄️ Freezer-Friendly  $
Budget-Friendly

### Ingredients

- 1 lb boneless, skinless chicken breast,
  diced
- 1 cup brown rice, cooked
- 1 cup black beans, rinsed and drained
- 1 cup corn kernels
- 1 cup diced tomatoes
- ½ cup shredded cheddar cheese
- 1 avocado, sliced
- 1 tbsp olive oil
- 1 tsp cumin, 1 tsp chili powder, salt &
  pepper to taste

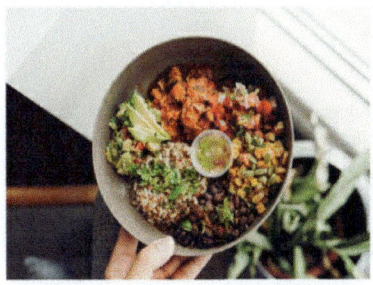

### Nutrition (per bowl)

- Calories: 480
- Protein: 42 g
- Carbs: 45 g (Fiber: 10 g)
- Fat: 15 g

### Directions

1. Heat olive oil in skillet; cook chicken with
   cumin, chili, salt, and pepper until done.
2. Assemble bowls with rice, beans, corn,
   tomatoes, and chicken.
3. Top with cheese and avocado slices.

### Storage & Prep

- Refrigerate up to 4 days.
- Store components separately for meal
  prep.

# Greek Chickpea Power Salad with Feta

Servings: 2  |  Prep Time: 10 min  |  Total Time: 10 min

Icons: 🌱 Plant-Based (with swaps)  ⏲ Under 30 Min  $ Budget-Friendly

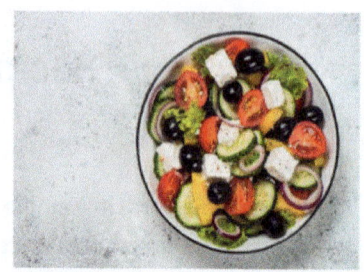

## Ingredients

- 1 can (15 oz) chickpeas, rinsed
- 1 cup cherry tomatoes, halved
- ½ cucumber, diced
- ¼ red onion, thinly sliced
- ¼ cup crumbled feta cheese
- 2 tbsp olive oil
- 1 tbsp lemon juice
- 1 tsp dried oregano
- Salt & pepper to taste

## Nutrition (per serving)

- Calories: 310
- Protein: 21 g
- Carbs: 34 g (Fiber: 9 g)
- Fat: 12 g

## Directions

1. Combine chickpeas, tomatoes, cucumber, and onion in a bowl.
2. Drizzle with olive oil, lemon juice, and oregano; toss well.
3. Top with feta and season with salt and pepper.

## Storage & Prep

- Refrigerate up to 3 days. Best eaten fresh.

# Lentil & Quinoa Buddha Bowl

Servings: 2  |  Prep Time: 15 min  |  Cook Time: 20 min  |  Total Time: 35 min

Icons: 🌱 Plant-Based  ❄ Freezer-Friendly  $ Budget-Friendly

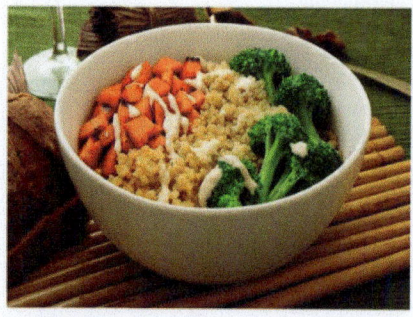

## Ingredients

- 1 cup cooked lentils
- 1 cup cooked quinoa
- 1 cup roasted broccoli
- 1 cup roasted sweet potatoes
- 2 tbsp tahini
- 1 tbsp lemon juice
- 1 tsp garlic powder
- 2 tbsp water (to thin)

## Nutrition (per serving)

- Calories: 420
- Protein: 31 g
- Carbs: 62 g (Fiber: 14 g)
- Fat: 12 g

## Directions

1. Divide lentils and quinoa into bowls.
2. Add roasted broccoli and sweet potatoes.
3. Whisk tahini, lemon juice, garlic powder, and water into dressing.
4. Drizzle over bowls before serving.

## Storage & Prep

- Refrigerate up to 4 days. Dressing keeps separately for 1 week.

# Asian Peanut Tofu & Edamame Bowl

Servings: 2  |  Prep Time: 15 min  |  Cook Time: 15 min  |  Total Time: 30 min
Icons: 🌱 Plant-Based  🍳 One-Pan  ❄️ Freezer-Friendly

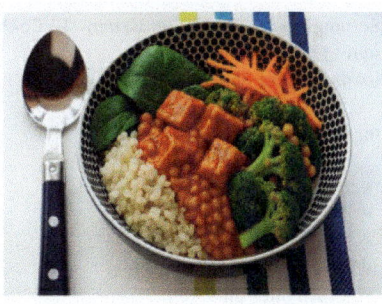

## Ingredients

- 14 oz firm tofu, cubed
- 1 cup shelled edamame
- 1 cup brown rice, cooked
- 1 cup steamed broccoli
- 2 tbsp peanut butter
- 1 tbsp soy sauce or tamari
- 1 tbsp rice vinegar
- 1 tsp sesame oil
- 1 tsp honey or maple syrup

### Nutrition (per serving)

- Calories: 460
- Protein: 35 g
- Carbs: 42 g (Fiber: 10 g)
- Fat: 16 g

## Directions

1. Heat skillet with sesame oil; cook tofu until golden.
2. Stir in peanut butter, soy sauce, vinegar, and honey; cook 2–3 minutes.
3. Assemble bowls with rice, tofu, edamame, and broccoli.

### Storage & Prep

- Refrigerate up to 4 days. Freeze tofu and rice separately for best texture.

# Creamy Tuna & White Bean Salad

Servings: 2  |  Prep Time: 10 min  |  Total Time: 10 min
Icons: ⏱ Under 30 Min  $ Budget-Friendly  ❄️ Freezer-Friendly (without greens)

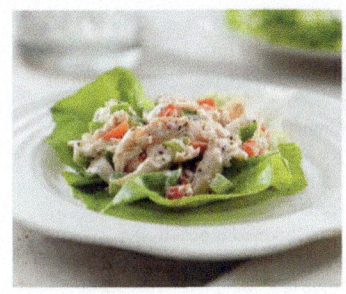

## Ingredients

- 1 can (5 oz) tuna in water, drained
- 1 cup canned white beans, rinsed
- 2 tbsp plain Greek yogurt
- 1 tbsp olive oil
- 1 tbsp lemon juice
- ½ cup chopped celery
- ¼ cup diced red onion
- Salt & pepper, to taste

### Nutrition (per serving)

- Calories: 280
- Protein: 29 g
- Carbs: 16 g (Fiber: 6 g)
- Fat: 10 g

## Directions

1. In a bowl, mash beans slightly with a fork.
2. Stir in tuna, yogurt, olive oil, lemon juice, celery, and onion.
3. Season with salt and pepper. Serve over greens or in wraps.

### Storage & Prep

- Refrigerate up to 3 days.
- Best prepped without greens until ready to serve.

# Spicy Shrimp & Quinoa Bowl

Servings: 2  |  Prep Time: 10 min  |  Cook Time: 10 min  |  Total Time: 20 min
Icons: 🔍 One-Pan  🕐 Under 30 Min

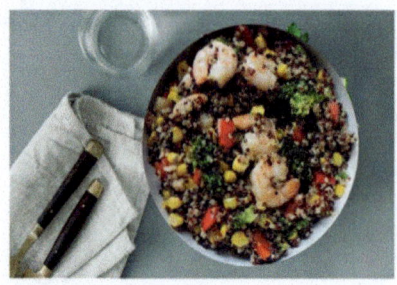

### Ingredients

- 8 oz shrimp, peeled and deveined
- 1 cup cooked quinoa
- 1 cup steamed broccoli
- ½ cup diced red bell pepper
- 1 tbsp olive oil
- 1 tsp chili powder
- 1 tsp paprika
- Juice of ½ lime

### Nutrition (per serving)

- Calories: 350
- Protein: 32 g
- Carbs: 32 g (Fiber: 6 g)
- Fat: 11 g

### Directions

1. Heat oil in skillet; season shrimp with chili and paprika.
2. Cook shrimp 2–3 minutes per side until pink.
3. Assemble bowls with quinoa, broccoli, peppers, and shrimp.
4. Drizzle with lime juice before serving.

### Storage & Prep

- Refrigerate up to 2 days. Best enjoyed fresh.

# Teriyaki Salmon Rice Bowl

Servings: 2  |  Prep Time: 10 min  |  Cook Time: 15 min  |  Total Time: 25 min
Icons: 🔍 One-Pan  ❄️ Freezer-Friendly

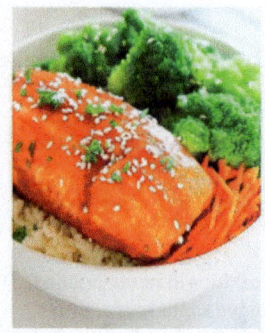

### Ingredients

- 2 salmon fillets (4 oz each)
- 2 cups cooked jasmine rice
- 1 cup steamed broccoli
- ½ cup shredded carrots
- 2 tbsp low-sodium teriyaki sauce
- 1 tsp sesame seeds

### Nutrition (per serving)

- Calories: 420
- Protein: 34 g
- Carbs: 36 g (Fiber: 5 g)
- Fat: 14 g

### Directions

1. Heat skillet over medium; cook salmon 4–5 minutes per side until flaky.
2. Drizzle with teriyaki sauce.
3. Assemble bowls with rice, salmon, broccoli, and carrots.
4. Sprinkle with sesame seeds before serving.

### Storage & Prep

- Refrigerate up to 3 days.
- Salmon can be frozen separately for up to 2 months.

# Mediterranean Turkey Meatball Bowl

Servings: 4  |  Prep Time: 15 min  |  Cook Time: 20 min  |  Total Time: 35 min
Icons: ❄ Freezer-Friendly  🍳 One-Pan

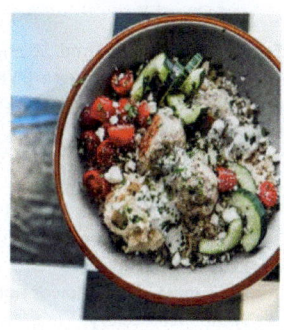

## Ingredients

- 1 lb lean ground turkey
- 1 egg
- ½ cup breadcrumbs (or oat flour for GF)
- 2 tsp garlic powder
- 1 tsp oregano
- 2 cups cooked farro or quinoa
- 1 cup cherry tomatoes
- 1 cup cucumber slices
- ¼ cup crumbled feta
- 2 tbsp tzatziki sauce

## Directions

1. Mix turkey, egg, breadcrumbs, garlic, and oregano. Form into 16 small meatballs.
2. Bake or pan-sear until fully cooked (about 15 minutes).
3. Assemble bowls with farro, meatballs, tomatoes, cucumber, feta, and tzatziki.

**Nutrition (per serving)**

- Calories: 430
- Protein: 39 g
- Carbs: 35 g (Fiber: 7 g)
- Fat: 15 g

**Storage & Prep**

- Refrigerate up to 4 days.
- Freeze meatballs up to 2 months.

# BBQ Chicken & Sweet Potato Bowl

Servings: 2  |  Prep Time: 10 min  |  Cook Time: 25 min  |  Total Time: 35 min
Icons: 🍳 One-Pan  ❄ Freezer-Friendly  $ Budget-Friendly

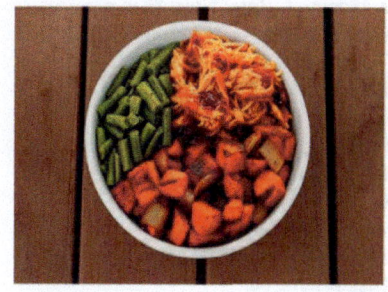

## Ingredients

- 8 oz cooked chicken breast, shredded
- 2 small sweet potatoes, diced
- 1 cup steamed green beans
- 2 tbsp BBQ sauce (low sugar if preferred)
- 1 tsp olive oil
- Salt & pepper, to taste

## Directions

1. Preheat oven to 400°F (200°C). Toss sweet potatoes with olive oil, salt, and pepper. Roast 20–25 minutes.
2. Heat chicken with BBQ sauce until warmed through.
3. Assemble bowls with sweet potatoes, chicken, and green beans.

**Nutrition (per serving)**

- Calories: 380
- Protein: 35 g
- Carbs: 38 g (Fiber: 7 g)
- Fat: 9 g

**Storage & Prep**

- Refrigerate up to 3 days.
- Freeze chicken separately for up to 2 months.

# Buffalo Chicken Quinoa Bowl

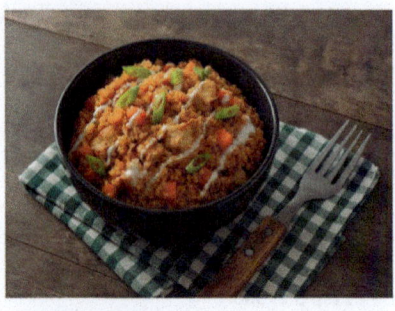

Servings: 2  |  Prep Time: 10 min  |  Cook Time: 15 min  |  Total Time: 25 min
Icons: 🔍 One-Pan  $ Budget-Friendly  ❄️ Freezer-Friendly

## Ingredients

- 8 oz cooked chicken breast, shredded
- 1 cup cooked quinoa
- 1 cup roasted cauliflower florets
- ½ cup diced celery
- 2 tbsp buffalo sauce
- 2 tbsp plain Greek yogurt (for drizzle)

## Directions

1. Toss shredded chicken with buffalo sauce.
2. Assemble bowls with quinoa, cauliflower, celery, and chicken.
3. Drizzle with Greek yogurt before serving.

### Nutrition (per serving)

- Calories: 370
- Protein: 36 g
- Carbs: 34 g (Fiber: 6 g)
- Fat: 10 g

### Storage & Prep

- Refrigerate up to 3 days.
- Freeze chicken separately for up to 2 months.

# Sesame Beef & Veggie Bowl

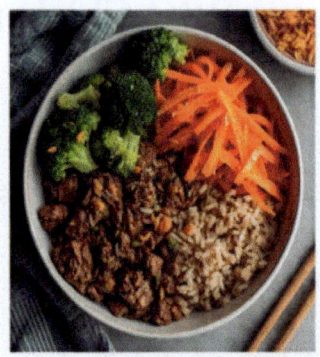

Servings: 2  |  Prep Time: 10 min  |  Cook Time: 15 min  |  Total Time: 25 min
Icons: 🔍 One-Pan  ❄️ Freezer-Friendly

## Ingredients

- 8 oz lean ground beef (90/10 or leaner)
- 1 cup brown rice, cooked
- 1 cup steamed broccoli
- ½ cup shredded carrots
- 1 tbsp low-sodium soy sauce or tamari
- 1 tsp sesame oil
- 1 tsp grated ginger
- 1 tsp sesame seeds

## Directions

1. Cook beef in skillet with sesame oil and ginger until browned.
2. Stir in soy sauce.
3. Assemble bowls with rice, beef, broccoli, and carrots.
4. Garnish with sesame seeds.

### Nutrition (per serving)

- Calories: 420
- Protein: 35 g
- Carbs: 34 g (Fiber: 5 g)
- Fat: 14 g

### Storage & Prep

- Refrigerate up to 4 days.
- Freeze beef mixture separately for up to 2 months.

# Caprese Chicken Pasta Salad

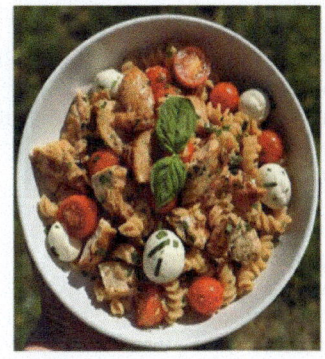

Servings: 4  |  Prep Time: 15 min  |  Cook Time: 10 min  |  Total Time: 25 min
Icons: ⏱ Under 30 Min   $ Budget-Friendly   ❄ Freezer-Friendly (without greens)

## Ingredients

- 8 oz whole wheat pasta, cooked
- 2 cups diced cooked chicken breast
- 1 cup cherry tomatoes, halved
- ½ cup fresh mozzarella balls
- ¼ cup fresh basil leaves, chopped
- 2 tbsp olive oil
- 1 tbsp balsamic vinegar
- Salt & pepper, to taste

**Nutrition (per serving)**

- Calories: 410
- Protein: 34 g
- Carbs: 36 g (Fiber: 7 g)
- Fat: 14 g

## Directions

1. Toss pasta, chicken, tomatoes, mozzarella, and basil in a bowl.
2. Drizzle with olive oil and balsamic vinegar.
3. Season with salt and pepper.

**Storage & Prep**

- Refrigerate up to 3 days.
- Best served chilled.

# Spicy Chickpea & Spinach Bowl

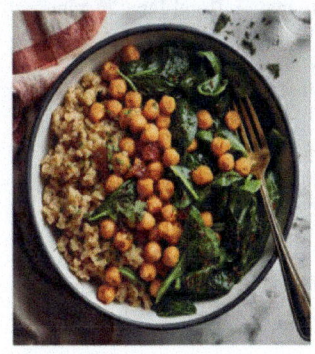

Servings: 2  |  Prep Time: 10 min  |  Cook Time: 10 min  |  Total Time: 20 min
Icons: 🌱 Plant-Based   🍳 One-Pan   $ Budget-Friendly

## Ingredients

- 1 can (15 oz) chickpeas, rinsed and drained
- 4 cups fresh spinach
- 1 cup cooked brown rice
- 1 tbsp olive oil
- 1 tsp smoked paprika
- ½ tsp cayenne pepper
- 1 tsp garlic powder

**Nutrition (per serving)**

- Calories: 360
- Protein: 24 g
- Carbs: 48 g (Fiber: 12 g)
- Fat: 10 g

## Directions

1. Heat oil in skillet; sauté chickpeas with spices 5 minutes.
2. Add spinach and cook until wilted.
3. Serve over rice.

**Storage & Prep**

- Refrigerate up to 3 days.
- Freezer-friendly up to 1 month (without spinach).

# Turkey Taco Salad Bowl

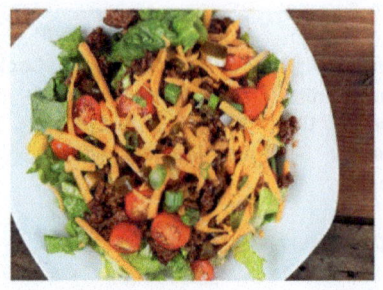

Servings: 2  |  Prep Time: 10 min  |  Cook Time: 15 min  |  Total Time: 25 min
Icons: 🔍 One-Pan  $ Budget-Friendly

### Ingredients
- 8 oz lean ground turkey
- 1 tsp chili powder
- 1 tsp cumin
- ½ tsp garlic powder
- 4 cups chopped romaine lettuce
- 1 cup cherry tomatoes, halved
- ½ cup black beans
- ¼ cup shredded cheddar cheese
- 2 tbsp salsa

### Directions
1. Cook turkey with chili powder, cumin, and garlic powder until browned.
2. Assemble bowls with lettuce, tomatoes, black beans, turkey, and cheese.
3. Top with salsa before serving.

**Nutrition (per serving)**

- Calories: 380
- Protein: 35 g
- Carbs: 28 g (Fiber: 8 g)
- Fat: 14 g

**Storage & Prep**

- Keep lettuce separate until ready to eat.
- Refrigerate turkey up to 4 days.

# Pesto Chicken & Farro Bowl

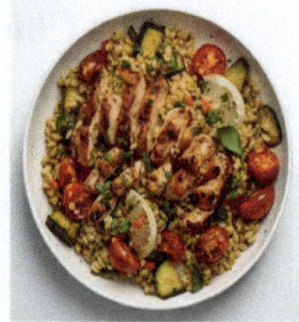

Servings: 2  |  Prep Time: 10 min  |  Cook Time: 15 min  |  Total Time: 25 min
Icons: 🔍 One-Pan  ❄ Freezer-Friendly

### Ingredients

- 8 oz grilled chicken breast, sliced
- 1 cup cooked farro
- 1 cup roasted zucchini and cherry tomatoes
- 2 tbsp basil pesto (store-bought or homemade)
- 1 tbsp grated Parmesan cheese

**Nutrition (per serving)**

- Calories: 400
- Protein: 37 g
- Carbs: 38 g (Fiber: 7 g)
- Fat: 13 g

**Storage & Prep**

- Refrigerate up to 3 days.
- Keep pesto separate until serving.

### Directions

1. Cook farro according to package instructions.
2. Roast zucchini and tomatoes until tender.
3. Assemble bowls with farro, chicken, veggies, and pesto.
4. Sprinkle with Parmesan before serving.

# Curry Lentil & Brown Rice Bowl

Servings: 2  |  Prep Time: 10 min  |  Cook Time: 20 min  |  Total Time: 30 min
Icons: 🌱 Plant-Based  🍳 One-Pan  $ Budget-Friendly

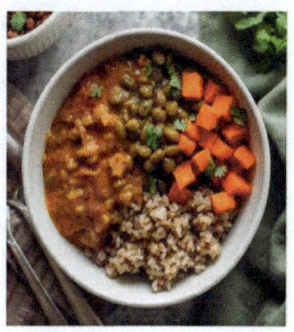

## Ingredients

- 1 cup cooked brown rice
- 1 cup cooked green lentils
- ½ cup diced carrots
- ½ cup peas
- 1 tbsp olive oil
- 1 tbsp curry powder
- ½ cup light coconut milk

**Nutrition (per serving)**

- Calories: 390
- Protein: 28 g
- Carbs: 55 g (Fiber: 12 g)
- Fat: 10 g

## Directions

1. Heat oil in skillet; sauté carrots and peas until tender.
2. Stir in lentils, curry powder, and coconut milk; simmer 5 minutes.
3. Serve over brown rice.

**Storage & Prep**

- Refrigerate up to 4 days.
- Freezer-friendly for up to 2 months.

# Garlic Herb Grilled Shrimp Bowl

Servings: 2  |  Prep Time: 10 min  |  Cook Time: 10 min  |  Total Time: 20 min
Icons: 🍳 One-Pan  ⏱ Under 30 Min

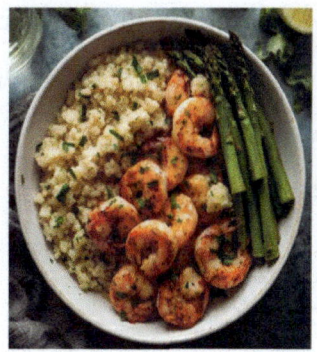

## Ingredients

- 8 oz shrimp, peeled and deveined
- 1 cup cooked couscous
- 1 cup steamed asparagus
- 1 tbsp olive oil
- 1 tsp garlic powder
- 1 tsp dried parsley
- Juice of ½ lemon

**Nutrition (per serving)**

- Calories: 350
- Protein: 32 g
- Carbs: 34 g (Fiber: 5 g)
- Fat: 10 g

## Directions

1. Heat skillet with olive oil; cook shrimp with garlic and parsley until pink.
2. Assemble bowls with couscous, asparagus, and shrimp.
3. Drizzle with lemon juice before serving.

**Storage & Prep**

- Refrigerate up to 2 days.
- Best enjoyed fresh.

# BBQ Tempeh Grain Bowl

Servings: 2  |  Prep Time: 10 min  |  Cook Time: 15 min  |  Total Time: 25 min
Icons: 🌱 Plant-Based  🔍 One-Pan  $ Budget-Friendly

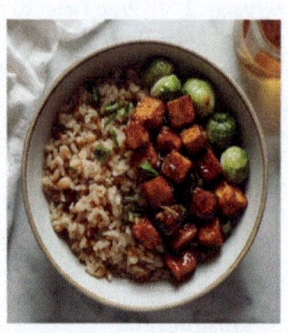

## Ingredients

- 8 oz tempeh, cubed
- 1 cup cooked barley or brown rice
- 1 cup roasted Brussels sprouts
- 2 tbsp BBQ sauce (low sugar if preferred)
- 1 tsp olive oil

## Directions

1. Heat skillet with olive oil; cook tempeh until golden.
2. Stir in BBQ sauce and simmer 2 minutes.
3. Assemble bowls with grain, Brussels sprouts, and tempeh.

### Nutrition (per serving)

- Calories: 380
- Protein: 28 g
- Carbs: 40 g (Fiber: 10 g)
- Fat: 12 g

### Storage & Prep

- Refrigerate up to 4 days.
- Freeze tempeh separately for up to 2 months.

# Mediterranean Salmon & Chickpea Bowl

Servings: 2  |  Prep Time: 10 min  |  Cook Time: 15 min  |  Total Time: 25 min
Icons: 🔍 One-Pan  ❄️ Freezer-Friendly

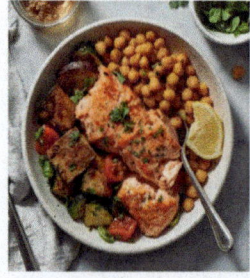

## Ingredients

- 2 salmon fillets (4 oz each)
- 1 cup cooked chickpeas
- 1 cup roasted eggplant and zucchini
- 1 tbsp olive oil
- 1 tsp oregano
- Juice of ½ lemon

## Directions

1. Heat skillet with olive oil; cook salmon until flaky.
2. Season chickpeas with oregano and roast with eggplant and zucchini until tender.
3. Assemble bowls with salmon, chickpeas, and roasted veggies.
4. Squeeze lemon juice before serving.

### Nutrition (per serving)

- Calories: 410
- Protein: 36 g
- Carbs: 32 g (Fiber: 9 g)
- Fat: 15 g

### Storage & Prep

- Refrigerate up to 3 days.
- Salmon and chickpeas freeze well for up to 2 months.

# Teriyaki Chicken & Veggie Bowl

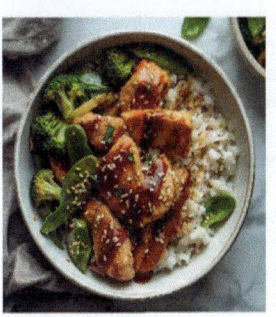

Servings: 2 | Prep Time: 10 min | Cook
Time: 15 min | Total Time: 25 min
Icons: 🔍 One-Pan ❄️ Freezer-Friendly $
Budget-Friendly

## Ingredients

- 8 oz chicken breast, diced
- 1 cup cooked jasmine rice
- 1 cup steamed broccoli
- ½ cup snap peas
- 2 tbsp low-sodium teriyaki sauce
- 1 tsp sesame seeds

### Nutrition (per serving)

- Calories: 380
- Protein: 36 g
- Carbs: 38 g (Fiber: 6 g)
- Fat: 8 g

## Directions

1. Heat skillet; cook chicken until browned.
2. Stir in teriyaki sauce and simmer 2 minutes.
3. Assemble bowls with rice, broccoli, snap peas, and chicken.
4. Sprinkle sesame seeds before serving.

### Storage & Prep

- Refrigerate up to 4 days.
- Freeze chicken and rice separately up to 2 months.

# Southwest Black Bean & Turkey Bowl

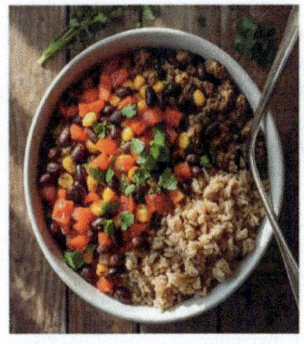

Servings: 2 | Prep Time: 10 min | Cook
Time: 15 min | Total Time: 25 min
Icons: 🔍 One-Pan $ Budget-Friendly

## Ingredients

- 8 oz lean ground turkey
- 1 cup cooked brown rice
- 1 cup black beans, rinsed
- 1 cup corn kernels
- ½ cup diced tomatoes
- 1 tsp cumin, 1 tsp chili powder

### Nutrition (per serving)

- Calories: 390
- Protein: 35 g
- Carbs: 40 g (Fiber: 10 g)
- Fat: 9 g

## Directions

1. Cook turkey with cumin and chili powder until browned.
2. Assemble bowls with rice, beans, corn, tomatoes, and turkey.

### Storage & Prep

- Refrigerate up to 4 days.
- Freezer-friendly up to 2 months.

# Thai Peanut Chicken Bowl

Servings: 2  |  Prep Time: 15 min  |  Cook
Time: 15 min  |  Total Time: 30 min
Icons: 🔍 One-Pan  ❄️ Freezer-Friendly

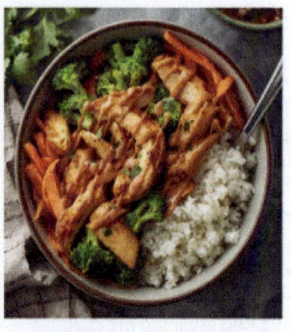

## Ingredients

- 8 oz chicken breast, sliced
- 1 cup cooked jasmine rice
- 1 cup steamed broccoli
- ½ cup shredded carrots
- 2 tbsp peanut butter
- 1 tbsp soy sauce
- 1 tbsp lime juice
- 1 tsp honey or maple syrup

## Nutrition (per serving)

- Calories: 420
- Protein: 38 g
- Carbs: 35 g (Fiber: 7 g)
- Fat: 13 g

## Directions

1. Cook chicken in skillet until browned.
2. Stir peanut butter, soy sauce, lime juice, and honey into a quick sauce.
3. Assemble bowls with rice, veggies, and chicken; drizzle sauce on top.

## Storage & Prep

- Refrigerate up to 3 days.
- Freeze chicken and sauce separately.

# Mediterranean Quinoa Power Bowl

Servings: 2  |  Prep Time: 10 min  |  Cook
Time: 15 min  |  Total Time: 25 min
Icons: 🌱 Plant-Based  $ Budget-Friendly

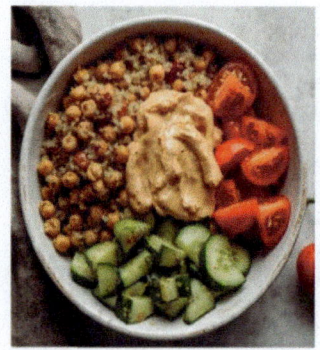

## Ingredients

- 1 cup cooked quinoa
- 1 cup roasted chickpeas
- ½ cup cucumber, diced
- ½ cup cherry tomatoes, halved
- 2 tbsp hummus
- 1 tbsp olive oil
- 1 tsp lemon juice

## Nutrition (per serving)

- Calories: 370
- Protein: 27 g
- Carbs: 44 g (Fiber: 11 g)
- Fat: 11 g

## Directions

1. Roast chickpeas with olive oil until crispy.
2. Assemble bowls with quinoa, chickpeas, cucumber, and tomatoes.
3. Top with hummus and lemon juice.

## Storage & Prep

- Refrigerate up to 4 days.
- Chickpeas can be roasted in advance and stored separately.

# Egg Roll in a Bowl

**Egg Roll in a Bowl**

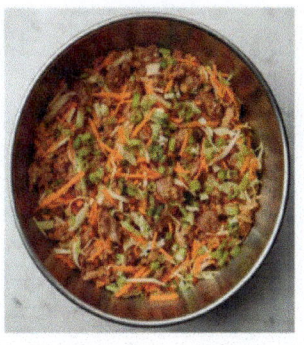

Servings: 2 | Prep Time: 10 min | Cook
Time: 15 min | Total Time: 25 min
Icons: 🔍 One-Pan $ Budget-Friendly

## Ingredients

- 8 oz lean ground pork or turkey
- 3 cups shredded cabbage
- 1 cup shredded carrots
- 2 green onions, sliced
- 1 tbsp low-sodium soy sauce
- 1 tsp sesame oil
- 1 tsp grated ginger

**Nutrition (per serving)**

- Calories: 360
- Protein: 34 g
- Carbs: 20 g (Fiber: 6 g)
- Fat: 14 g

## Directions

1. Heat sesame oil in skillet; cook ground meat until browned.
2. Add cabbage, carrots, soy sauce, and ginger. Cook until veggies are tender.
3. Garnish with green onions.

**Storage & Prep**

- Refrigerate up to 4 days.
- Freezer-friendly for up to 2 months.

# Chapter 6

# Dinners Made Simple

✦

Dinner is often the meal where healthy eating falls apart—long workdays, busy evenings, and limited energy make takeout tempting. This chapter brings you more than 30 high-protein dinners that are fast, flexible, and family-friendly.

You'll find:

- **Sheet-pan meals** that cook everything at once with almost no cleanup.

- **One-pot and skillet dinners** packed with flavor but light on effort.

- **Slow cooker and Instant Pot favorites** that do the work for you.

- **Better-than-takeout recipes** that satisfy cravings with lean proteins and nutrient-rich ingredients.

- **Balanced bowls and hearty classics** designed to keep you full and fueled until morning.

Each recipe is designed with protein front and center, paired with vegetables and smart carbs to create complete meals. With simple prep, minimal cleanup, and make-ahead options, these dinners prove that eating high-protein at night doesn't have to be complicated—or boring.

# Recipe Icons Guide

🔍 **One-Pan**
Cook the whole meal in a single pan —
less cleanup, more convenience.

❄️ **Freezer-Friendly**
Can be stored in the freezer for later;
reheats well.

$ **Budget-Friendly**
Costs under $4 per serving with
common ingredients.

⏱️ **Under 30 Minutes**
From prep to plate in half an hour or
less.

⭐ **30+ g Protein**
Each serving delivers at least 30 grams
of protein.

🌱 **Plant-Based**
Fully vegetarian or vegan protein
sources.

# Sheet-Pan Lemon Herb Salmon with Veggies

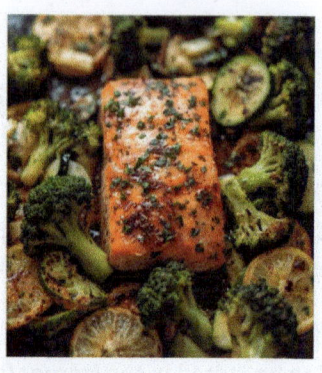

Servings: 2  |  Prep Time: 10 min  |  Cook Time: 15 min  |  Total Time: 25 min
Icons: 🔍 One-Pan  ⏱ Under 30 Min  ❄ Freezer-Friendly

## Ingredients

- 2 salmon fillets (4 oz each)
- 1 cup broccoli florets
- 1 cup zucchini slices
- 1 tbsp olive oil
- 1 tsp dried oregano
- Juice of 1 lemon
- Salt & pepper, to taste

**Nutrition (per serving)**

- Calories: 370
- Protein: 34 g
- Carbs: 12 g (Fiber: 4 g)
- Fat: 20 g

## Directions

1. Preheat oven to 400°F (200°C). Line sheet-pan with parchment.
2. Arrange salmon and veggies. Drizzle with olive oil, lemon juice, oregano, salt, and pepper.
3. Roast 12–15 minutes until salmon flakes easily and veggies are tender.

**Storage & Prep**

- Refrigerate up to 3 days.
- Freeze salmon separately up to 2 months.

# Garlic Butter Chicken & Broccoli Skillet

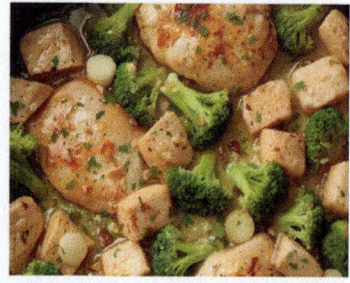

Servings: 2  |  Prep Time: 10 min  |  Cook Time: 15 min  |  Total Time: 25 min
Icons: 🔍 One-Pan  ⏱ Under 30 Min  $ Budget-Friendly

## Ingredients

- 8 oz chicken breast, cubed
- 2 cups broccoli florets
- 2 tbsp butter
- 2 garlic cloves, minced
- ½ tsp paprika
- Salt & pepper, to taste

**Nutrition (per serving)**

- Calories: 360
- Protein: 38 g
- Carbs: 10 g (Fiber: 4 g)
- Fat: 18 g

## Directions

1. Melt butter in skillet; sauté garlic 1 minute.
2. Add chicken, season with paprika, salt, and pepper; cook until golden.
3. Stir in broccoli; cook until tender but crisp.

**Storage & Prep**

- Refrigerate up to 4 days.
- Best reheated in skillet to keep broccoli crisp.

# Slow Cooker Pulled BBQ Turkey

Servings: 4  |  Prep Time: 10 min  |  Cook Time: 6 hrs (slow cooker)  |  Total Time: 6 hrs+

Icons: ❄ Freezer-Friendly  $ Budget-Friendly

### Ingredients

- 1 lb turkey breast (boneless)
- ½ cup low-sugar BBQ sauce
- 1 tsp smoked paprika
- ½ tsp garlic powder
- ½ cup chicken broth

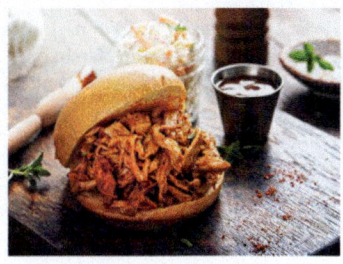

### Directions

1. Place turkey, broth, paprika, and garlic in slow cooker.
2. Cook on low 6–7 hours or high 3–4 hours until tender.
3. Shred turkey with forks and toss with BBQ sauce.

### Nutrition (per serving)

- Calories: 280
- Protein: 35 g
- Carbs: 10 g (Fiber: 1 g)
- Fat: 9 g

### Storage & Prep

- Refrigerate up to 4 days.
- Freeze shredded turkey with sauce up to 2 months.

# One-Pot Beef & Lentil Chili

Servings: 4  |  Prep Time: 15 min  |  Cook Time: 30 min  |  Total Time: 45 min

Icons: 🔍 One-Pan  ❄ Freezer-Friendly  $ Budget-Friendly

### Ingredients

- 1 lb lean ground beef
- 1 cup cooked lentils
- 1 can (15 oz) diced tomatoes
- 1 can (15 oz) kidney beans, rinsed
- 1 onion, diced
- 2 garlic cloves, minced
- 1 tbsp chili powder
- 1 tsp cumin
- 1 cup beef broth

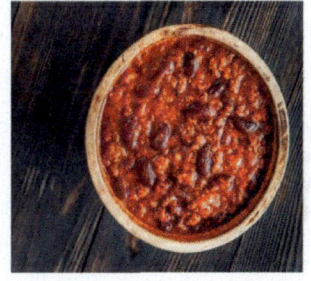

### Nutrition (per serving)

- Calories: 420
- Protein: 37 g
- Carbs: 40 g (Fiber: 12 g)
- Fat: 12 g

### Directions

1. Brown beef with onion and garlic in pot.
2. Stir in lentils, beans, tomatoes, broth, and spices.
3. Simmer 20–25 minutes until thick.

### Storage & Prep

- Refrigerate up to 5 days.
- Freezer-friendly for up to 2 months.

# High-Protein Shrimp Fried "Rice" (Cauliflower Base)

Servings: 2  |  Prep Time: 10 min  |  Cook Time: 10 min  |  Total Time: 20 min
Icons: 🔍 One-Pan  ⏱ Under 30 Min

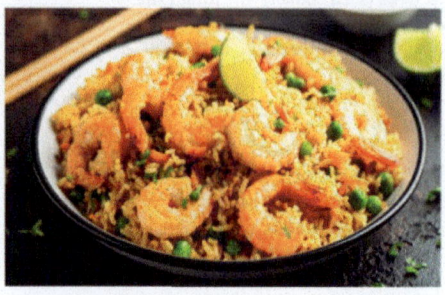

### Ingredients

- 8 oz shrimp, peeled and deveined
- 2 cups riced cauliflower
- 1 cup mixed vegetables (peas, carrots, corn)
- 2 large eggs, whisked
- 1 tbsp soy sauce (low sodium)
- 1 tsp sesame oil

### Directions

1. Heat sesame oil in skillet; cook shrimp until pink. Remove and set aside.
2. Add cauliflower rice and mixed veggies; sauté 3–4 minutes.
3. Push to side; scramble eggs, then stir everything together.
4. Add soy sauce and shrimp; cook 1 minute.

### Nutrition (per serving)

- Calories: 310
- Protein: 32 g
- Carbs: 16 g (Fiber: 6 g)
- Fat: 12 g

### Storage & Prep

- Refrigerate up to 3 days.
- Best reheated in skillet, not microwave, to avoid sogginess.

# Teriyaki Chicken Stir-Fry

Servings: 2  |  Prep Time: 10 min  |  Cook Time: 15 min  |  Total Time: 25 min
Icons: 🔍 One-Pan  ⏱ Under 30 Min  $ Budget-Friendly

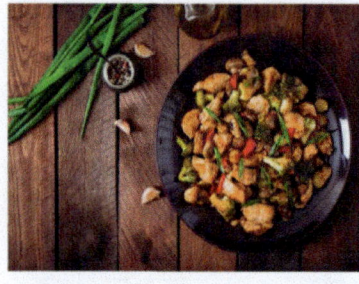

### Ingredients

- 8 oz chicken breast, sliced thin
- 2 cups mixed stir-fry vegetables (broccoli, snap peas, bell peppers)
- 1 cup cooked brown rice
- 2 tbsp low-sodium teriyaki sauce
- 1 tsp sesame oil

### Directions

1. Heat sesame oil in skillet; cook chicken until browned.
2. Add vegetables; stir-fry 5 minutes until crisp-tender.
3. Stir in teriyaki sauce; cook 1–2 minutes.
4. Serve over rice.

### Nutrition (per serving)

- Calories: 390
- Protein: 37 g
- Carbs: 40 g (Fiber: 6 g)
- Fat: 10 g

### Storage & Prep

- Refrigerate up to 4 days.
- Freeze chicken/veggie mix separately from rice.

# Stuffed Peppers with Quinoa & Ground Turkey

Servings: 4  |  Prep Time: 15 min  |  Cook Time: 35 min  |  Total Time: 50 min
Icons: ❄ Freezer-Friendly   $ Budget-Friendly

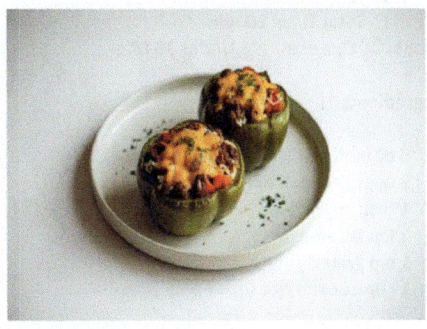

## Ingredients

- 4 large bell peppers, tops removed
- 1 lb ground turkey
- 1 cup cooked quinoa
- 1 cup diced tomatoes
- ½ cup shredded mozzarella cheese
- 1 tsp garlic powder, 1 tsp oregano
- Salt & pepper, to taste

## Directions

1. Preheat oven to 375°F (190°C).
2. Cook turkey with garlic powder, oregano, salt, and pepper until browned.
3. Stir in quinoa and tomatoes.
4. Stuff peppers with mixture, top with cheese, and bake 30–35 minutes.

**Nutrition (per pepper)**
- Calories: 340
- Protein: 33 g
- Carbs: 28 g (Fiber: 6 g)
- Fat: 11 g

**Storage & Prep**
- Refrigerate up to 4 days.
- Freeze individually wrapped peppers up to 2 months.

# Honey Garlic Glazed Salmon with Green Beans

Servings: 2  |  Prep Time: 10 min  |  Cook Time: 15 min  |  Total Time: 25 min
Icons: 🔍 One-Pan   ⏱ Under 30 Min

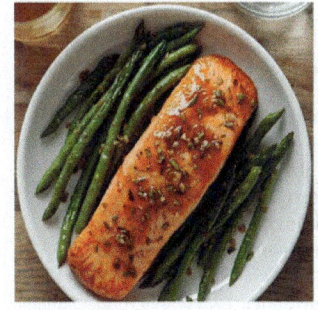

## Ingredients

- 2 salmon fillets (4 oz each)
- 2 cups green beans, trimmed
- 1 tbsp olive oil
- 1 tbsp soy sauce
- 1 tbsp honey
- 2 garlic cloves, minced

## Directions

1. Heat olive oil in skillet; add garlic and cook 1 minute.
2. Stir in soy sauce and honey.
3. Add salmon fillets; cook 4–5 minutes per side, basting with glaze.
4. Add green beans to pan; sauté until tender-crisp.

**Nutrition (per serving)**

- Calories: 370
- Protein: 34 g
- Carbs: 16 g (Fiber: 4 g)
- Fat: 18 g

**Storage & Prep**

- Refrigerate up to 3 days.
- Salmon freezes well up to 2 months.

# Beef & Broccoli Stir-Fry

Servings: 2 | Prep Time: 10 min | Cook Time: 10 min | Total Time: 20 min
Icons: 🔍 One-Pan 🕐 Under 30 Min

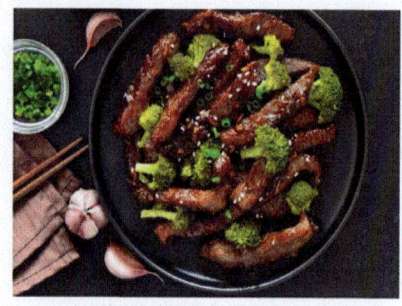

### Ingredients

- 8 oz lean beef sirloin, sliced thin
- 2 cups broccoli florets
- 1 tbsp soy sauce
- 1 tsp sesame oil
- 1 tsp grated ginger
- 1 cup cooked rice (optional)

**Nutrition (per serving, without rice)**

- Calories: 300
- Protein: 35 g
- Carbs: 10 g (Fiber: 3 g)
- Fat: 14 g

### Directions

1. Heat sesame oil in skillet; cook beef 2–3 minutes until browned.
2. Add broccoli, ginger, and soy sauce; stir-fry 5 minutes.
3. Serve as-is or over rice.

**Storage & Prep**

- Refrigerate up to 3 days.
- Best reheated quickly in skillet.

# One-Pot Creamy Tuscan Chicken

Servings: 4 | Prep Time: 15 min | Cook Time: 25 min | Total Time: 40 min
Icons: 🔍 One-Pan ❄️ Freezer-Friendly

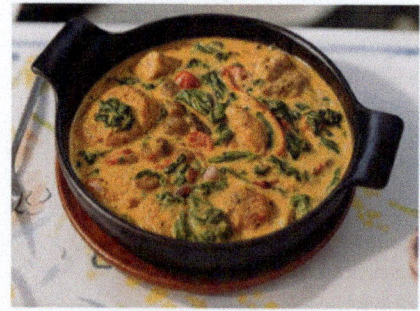

### Ingredients

- 1 lb chicken breast, cubed
- 1 tbsp olive oil
- 2 garlic cloves, minced
- 1 cup cherry tomatoes, halved
- 2 cups spinach
- ½ cup light cream or evaporated milk
- ¼ cup grated Parmesan cheese
- 1 tsp Italian seasoning

**Nutrition (per serving)**

- Calories: 400
- Protein: 39 g
- Carbs: 10 g (Fiber: 3 g)
- Fat: 20 g

### Directions

1. Heat olive oil in skillet; cook chicken until browned.
2. Add garlic and tomatoes; cook 3 minutes.
3. Stir in cream, Parmesan, and Italian seasoning. Simmer until thickened.
4. Add spinach; cook until wilted.

**Storage & Prep**

- Refrigerate up to 4 days.
- Freeze without spinach for best texture (add fresh when reheating).

# Turkey Meatloaf with Roasted Veggies

Servings: 4 | Prep Time: 15 min | Cook Time: 45 min | Total Time: 1 hr
Icons: ❄ Freezer-Friendly $ Budget-Friendly

## Ingredients

- 1 lb lean ground turkey
- 1 egg
- ½ cup breadcrumbs (or oat flour for GF)
- ½ cup diced onion
- 1 tsp garlic powder
- 1 tsp oregano
- 1 tbsp ketchup (plus extra for topping)
- 2 cups mixed roasted vegetables (carrots, zucchini, broccoli)

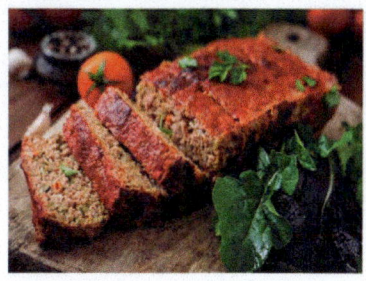

## Directions

1. Preheat oven to 375°F (190°C).
2. Mix turkey, egg, breadcrumbs, onion, garlic powder, oregano, and ketchup.
3. Shape into loaf, place in baking dish, and spread extra ketchup on top.
4. Bake 40–45 minutes until cooked through. Serve with roasted veggies.

**Nutrition (per serving)**

- Calories: 380
- Protein: 36 g
- Carbs: 26 g (Fiber: 5 g)
- Fat: 13 g

**Storage & Prep**

- Refrigerate up to 4 days.
- Freeze individual slices up to 2 months.

# Cajun Shrimp & Sausage Skillet

Cajun Shrimp & Sausage Skillet

Servings: 3 | Prep Time: 10 min | Cook Time: 15 min | Total Time: 25 min
Icons: 🔍 One-Pan ⏱ Under 30 Min

## Ingredients

- 8 oz shrimp, peeled and deveined
- 6 oz chicken sausage, sliced
- 1 red bell pepper, sliced
- 1 zucchini, sliced
- 1 tbsp olive oil
- 1 tsp Cajun seasoning

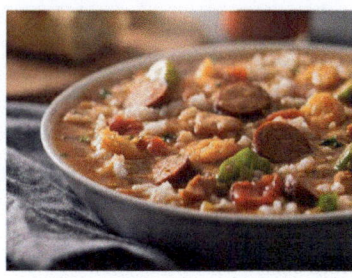

**Nutrition (per serving)**

- Calories: 340
- Protein: 32 g
- Carbs: 12 g (Fiber: 3 g)
- Fat: 18 g

**Storage & Prep**

- Refrigerate up to 3 days.
- Best reheated in skillet to keep shrimp tender.

## Directions

1. Heat olive oil in skillet; cook sausage until browned.
2. Add shrimp and Cajun seasoning; cook until shrimp turn pink.
3. Stir in bell pepper and zucchini; sauté until tender-crisp.

# Baked Lemon Garlic Cod with Asparagus

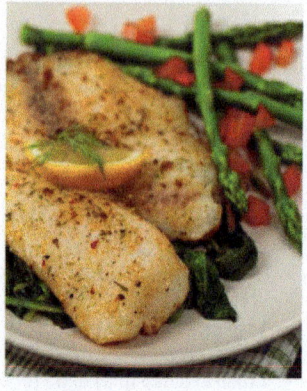

Servings: 2 | Prep Time: 10 min | Cook
Time: 15 min | Total Time: 25 min
Icons: 🔍 One-Pan ⏲ Under 30 Min

**Ingredients**

- 2 cod fillets (4 oz each)
- 2 cups asparagus spears
- 1 tbsp olive oil
- 2 garlic cloves, minced
- Juice of ½ lemon
- Salt & pepper, to taste

**Directions**

1. Preheat oven to 400°F (200°C).
2. Arrange cod and asparagus on a baking sheet.
3. Drizzle with olive oil, garlic, lemon juice, salt, and pepper.
4. Bake 12–15 minutes until fish flakes easily.

**Nutrition (per serving)**

- Calories: 280
- Protein: 33 g
- Carbs: 8 g (Fiber: 3 g)
- Fat: 12 g

**Storage & Prep**

- Refrigerate up to 3 days.
- Not ideal for freezing; enjoy fresh.

# One-Pot Chicken & Chickpea Curry

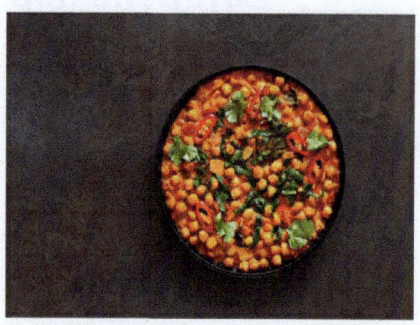

Servings: 4 | Prep Time: 15 min | Cook
Time: 25 min | Total Time: 40 min
Icons: 🔍 One-Pan ❄ Freezer-Friendly

**Ingredients**

- 1 lb chicken breast, cubed
- 1 can (15 oz) chickpeas, rinsed
- 1 can (15 oz) diced tomatoes
- 1 cup light coconut milk
- 1 onion, diced
- 2 tbsp curry powder
- 1 tbsp olive oil
- Salt & pepper, to taste

**Directions**

1. Heat olive oil in pot; cook onion until softened.
2. Add chicken; cook until browned.
3. Stir in chickpeas, tomatoes, coconut milk, and curry powder.
4. Simmer 20 minutes until thickened.

**Nutrition (per serving)**

- Calories: 420
- Protein: 39 g
- Carbs: 30 g (Fiber: 8 g)
- Fat: 16 g

**Storage & Prep**

- Refrigerate up to 4 days.
- Freezer-friendly up to 2 months.

# Beef & Sweet Potato Hash

Servings: 3  |  Prep Time: 10 min  |  Cook Time: 20 min  |  Total Time: 30 min
Icons: 🔍 One-Pan  ⏱ Under 30 Min  $ Budget-Friendly

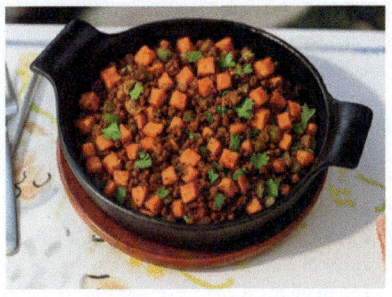

### Ingredients

- 12 oz lean ground beef
- 2 medium sweet potatoes, diced
- 1 bell pepper, diced
- 1 onion, diced
- 1 tbsp olive oil
- 1 tsp smoked paprika
- Salt & pepper, to taste

### Nutrition (per serving)

- Calories: 390
- Protein: 34 g
- Carbs: 35 g (Fiber: 7 g)
- Fat: 14 g

### Directions

1. Heat olive oil in skillet; sauté sweet potatoes until golden.
2. Add onion and bell pepper; cook until softened.
3. Stir in beef, paprika, salt, and pepper; cook until beef is browned.

### Storage & Prep

- Refrigerate up to 4 days.
- Freezer-friendly for up to 2 months.

# BBQ Chicken Sheet-Pan Dinner

Servings: 4  |  Prep Time: 10 min  |  Cook Time: 25 min  |  Total Time: 35 min
Icons: 🔍 One-Pan  ❄ Freezer-Friendly  $ Budget-Friendly

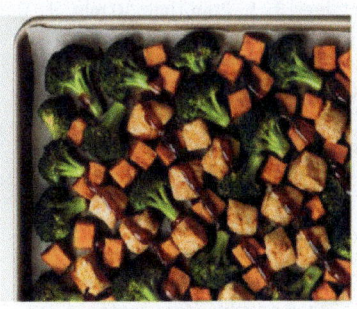

### Ingredients

- 1 lb chicken breast, cubed
- 2 cups broccoli florets
- 2 cups diced sweet potatoes
- 2 tbsp olive oil
- ¼ cup BBQ sauce (low sugar if preferred)
- Salt & pepper, to taste

### Nutrition (per serving)

- Calories: 370
- Protein: 36 g
- Carbs: 32 g (Fiber: 7 g)
- Fat: 11 g

### Directions

1. Preheat oven to 400°F (200°C).
2. Toss chicken and veggies with olive oil, salt, and pepper.
3. Spread on sheet-pan and roast 20–25 minutes until chicken is cooked and potatoes are tender.
4. Toss with BBQ sauce before serving.

### Storage & Prep

- Refrigerate up to 4 days.
- Freeze chicken separately up to 2 months.

# Lemon Garlic Shrimp Zoodles

Servings: 2 | Prep Time: 10 min | Cook Time: 10 min | Total Time: 20 min
Icons: 🔍 One-Pan  ⏱ Under 30 Min

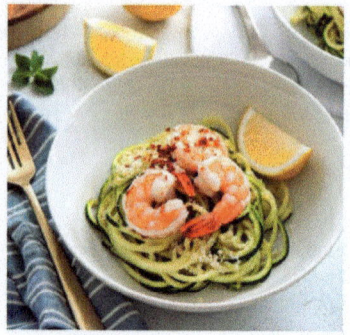

### Ingredients

- 8 oz shrimp, peeled and deveined
- 2 medium zucchini, spiralized
- 2 garlic cloves, minced
- Juice of 1 lemon
- 1 tbsp olive oil
- 2 tbsp Parmesan cheese (optional)

### Directions

1. Heat olive oil in skillet; cook garlic 1 minute.
2. Add shrimp; cook 2–3 minutes per side until pink.
3. Toss in zucchini noodles and lemon juice; cook 2–3 minutes until just tender.
4. Top with Parmesan if desired.

### Nutrition (per serving)

- Calories: 270
- Protein: 31 g
- Carbs: 10 g (Fiber: 3 g)
- Fat: 12 g

### Storage & Prep

- Best enjoyed fresh.
- Refrigerate up to 2 days (zoodles soften quickly).

# Greek Turkey Skillet with Feta

Servings: 3 | Prep Time: 10 min | Cook Time: 15 min | Total Time: 25 min
Icons: 🔍 One-Pan  ⏱ Under 30 Min  $ Budget-Friendly

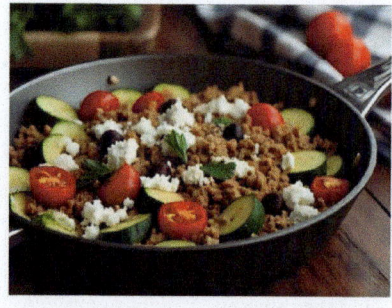

### Ingredients

- 12 oz lean ground turkey
- 1 cup diced zucchini
- 1 cup cherry tomatoes, halved
- ½ cup kalamata olives, sliced
- 2 tbsp crumbled feta cheese
- 1 tsp oregano
- 1 tbsp olive oil

### Nutrition (per serving)

- Calories: 320
- Protein: 33 g
- Carbs: 12 g (Fiber: 4 g)
- Fat: 15 g

### Directions

1. Heat olive oil in skillet; cook turkey with oregano until browned.
2. Add zucchini and tomatoes; cook until softened.
3. Stir in olives and sprinkle with feta before serving.

### Storage & Prep

- Refrigerate up to 4 days.
- Freeze turkey mixture without feta for up to 2 months.

# One-Pot Lentil & Spinach Stew

Servings: 4  |  Prep Time: 10 min  |  Cook Time: 25 min  |  Total Time: 35 min
Icons: 🌱 Plant-Based  🍳 One-Pan  ❄️ Freezer-Friendly

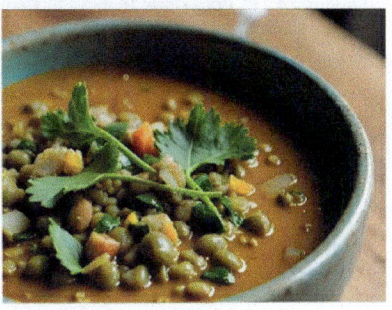

## Ingredients

- 1 cup green lentils, rinsed
- 4 cups vegetable broth
- 2 cups spinach
- 1 carrot, diced
- 1 onion, diced
- 2 garlic cloves, minced
- 1 tsp cumin
- 1 tsp smoked paprika

**Nutrition (per serving)**

- Calories: 310
- Protein: 24 g
- Carbs: 45 g (Fiber: 13 g)
- Fat: 5 g

## Directions

1. Heat onion, garlic, and carrot in pot 3–4 minutes.
2. Stir in lentils, broth, cumin, and paprika. Simmer 20–25 minutes until lentils are tender.
3. Add spinach and stir until wilted.

**Storage & Prep**

- Refrigerate up to 5 days.
- Freeze up to 2 months.

# Balsamic Glazed Chicken with Brussels Sprouts

Servings: 2  |  Prep Time: 10 min  |  Cook Time: 20 min  |  Total Time: 30 min
Icons: 🍳 One-Pan  🕐 Under 30 Min  ❄️ Freezer-Friendly

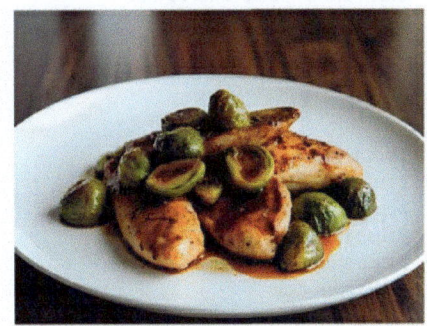

## Ingredients

- 8 oz chicken breast, halved
- 2 cups Brussels sprouts, halved
- 1 tbsp olive oil
- 2 tbsp balsamic vinegar
- 1 tsp honey
- Salt & pepper, to taste

**Nutrition (per serving)**

- Calories: 360
- Protein: 35 g
- Carbs: 18 g (Fiber: 6 g)
- Fat: 14 g

## Directions

1. Heat olive oil in skillet; cook chicken until golden. Remove and set aside.
2. Add Brussels sprouts; sauté until browned.
3. Stir in balsamic vinegar and honey; return chicken to pan.
4. Simmer until sauce thickens and chicken is fully cooked.

**Storage & Prep**

- Refrigerate up to 4 days.
- Freeze chicken separately for up to 2 months.

# Chicken Parmesan Skillet

Servings: 4 | Prep Time: 15 min | Cook Time: 25 min | Total Time: 40 min
Icons: 🔍 One-Pan ❄️ Freezer-Friendly

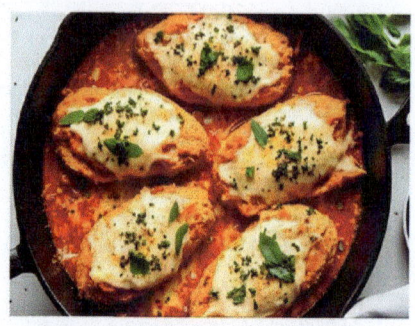

### Ingredients

- 1 lb chicken breast, cutlets or cubes
- 1 cup marinara sauce (low sugar)
- ½ cup shredded mozzarella cheese
- ¼ cup grated Parmesan cheese
- 1 tbsp olive oil
- 1 tsp Italian seasoning

### Directions

1. Heat olive oil in skillet; cook chicken with Italian seasoning until browned.
2. Pour marinara sauce over chicken; simmer 10 minutes.
3. Sprinkle mozzarella and Parmesan on top; cover until melted.

### Nutrition (per serving)

- Calories: 360
- Protein: 38 g
- Carbs: 10 g (Fiber: 3 g)
- Fat: 16 g

### Storage & Prep

- Refrigerate up to 4 days.
- Freeze chicken in sauce up to 2 months.

# Spicy Tofu & Vegetable Stir-Fry

Servings: 2 | Prep Time: 10 min | Cook Time: 15 min | Total Time: 25 min
Icons: 🌱 Plant-Based 🔍 One-Pan ⏱️ Under 30 Min

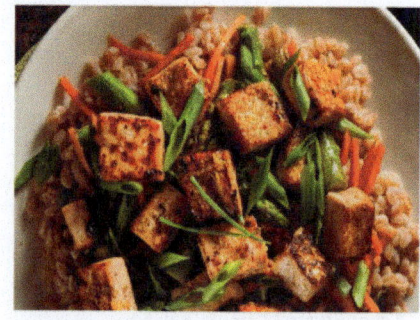

### Ingredients

- 14 oz firm tofu, cubed
- 2 cups mixed vegetables (broccoli, peppers, carrots)
- 2 tbsp soy sauce
- 1 tbsp sriracha or chili garlic sauce
- 1 tsp sesame oil
- 1 tsp grated ginger

### Directions

1. Heat sesame oil in skillet; cook tofu until golden.
2. Add vegetables, soy sauce, and ginger; stir-fry 5–6 minutes.
3. Drizzle with sriracha before serving.

### Nutrition (per serving)

- Calories: 320
- Protein: 28 g
- Carbs: 20 g (Fiber: 6 g)
- Fat: 14 g

### Storage & Prep

- Refrigerate up to 4 days.
- Best reheated in skillet, not microwave.

# Rosemary Garlic Pork Tenderloin

Servings: 4 | Prep Time: 15 min | Cook Time: 25 min | Total Time: 40 min
Icons: ❄ Freezer-Friendly  $ Budget-Friendly

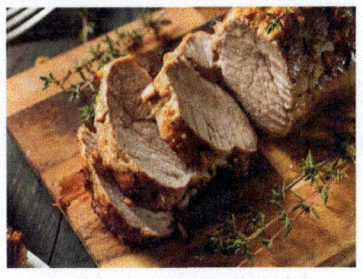

### Ingredients

- 1 lb pork tenderloin
- 1 tbsp olive oil
- 2 garlic cloves, minced
- 1 tsp rosemary
- 1 tsp thyme
- Salt & pepper, to taste

### Directions

1. Preheat oven to 400°F (200°C).
2. Rub tenderloin with olive oil, garlic, rosemary, thyme, salt, and pepper.
3. Roast 25–30 minutes until internal temperature reaches 145°F (63°C).
4. Rest 5 minutes before slicing.

**Nutrition (per serving)**

- Calories: 300
- Protein: 34 g
- Carbs: 4 g (Fiber: 1 g)
- Fat: 15 g

**Storage & Prep**

- Refrigerate up to 4 days.
- Freeze cooked slices up to 2 months.

# Chickpea & Spinach Stuffed Sweet Potatoes

Servings: 2 | Prep Time: 10 min | Cook Time: 40 min | Total Time: 50 min
Icons: 🌱 Plant-Based  $ Budget-Friendly

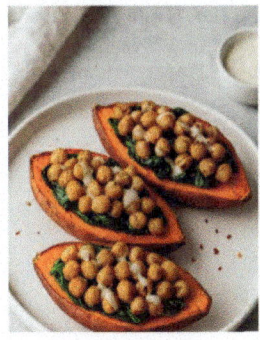

### Ingredients

- 2 medium sweet potatoes
- 1 cup canned chickpeas, rinsed
- 2 cups spinach
- 1 tbsp olive oil
- 1 tsp smoked paprika
- 1 tbsp tahini (optional drizzle)

### Directions

1. Preheat oven to 400°F (200°C). Bake sweet potatoes 40 minutes until tender.
2. Heat olive oil in skillet; sauté chickpeas with paprika, then stir in spinach until wilted.
3. Slice sweet potatoes open and stuff with chickpea-spinach mix.
4. Drizzle with tahini if desired.

**Nutrition (per serving)**

- Calories: 360
- Protein: 22 g
- Carbs: 56 g (Fiber: 12 g)
- Fat: 9 g

**Storage & Prep**

- Refrigerate up to 4 days.
- Freeze filling separately for up to 2 months.

# Asian Beef & Cabbage Stir-Fry

Servings: 3  |  Prep Time: 10 min  |  Cook Time: 15 min  |  Total Time: 25 min
Icons: 🔍 One-Pan  ⏱ Under 30 Min  $ Budget-Friendly

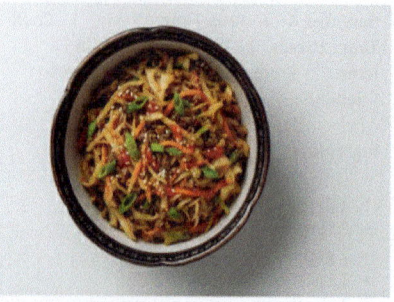

### Ingredients

- 12 oz lean ground beef
- 3 cups shredded cabbage
- 1 carrot, shredded
- 2 tbsp soy sauce
- 1 tsp sesame oil
- 1 tsp garlic powder
- ½ tsp chili flakes (optional)

### Directions

1. Heat sesame oil in skillet; cook beef with garlic until browned.
2. Add cabbage, carrot, soy sauce, and chili flakes.
3. Stir-fry until cabbage softens but remains slightly crisp.

### Nutrition (per serving)

- Calories: 340
- Protein: 32 g
- Carbs: 14 g (Fiber: 4 g)
- Fat: 16 g

### Storage & Prep

- Refrigerate up to 4 days.
- Freeze beef mixture separately for up to 2 months.

# One-Pot Turkey & Vegetable Soup

Servings: 4  |  Prep Time: 15 min  |  Cook Time: 30 min  |  Total Time: 45 min
Icons: 🔍 One-Pan  ❄ Freezer-Friendly  $ Budget-Friendly

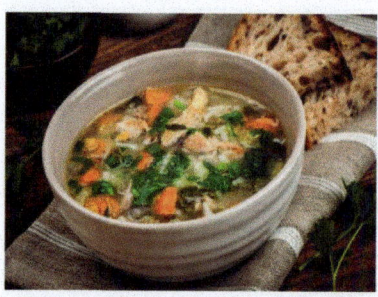

### Ingredients

- 1 lb ground turkey
- 1 onion, diced
- 2 carrots, diced
- 2 celery stalks, diced
- 1 zucchini, diced
- 1 can (15 oz) diced tomatoes
- 4 cups chicken broth
- 1 tsp oregano, 1 tsp garlic powder

### Directions

1. Brown turkey in large pot. Add onion, carrots, and celery; sauté 5 minutes.
2. Stir in zucchini, tomatoes, broth, and spices.
3. Simmer 25–30 minutes until vegetables are tender.

### Nutrition (per serving)

- Calories: 310
- Protein: 32 g
- Carbs: 22 g (Fiber: 5 g)
- Fat: 11 g

### Storage & Prep

- Refrigerate up to 5 days.
- Freeze up to 2 months.

# Lemon Dill Salmon with Quinoa

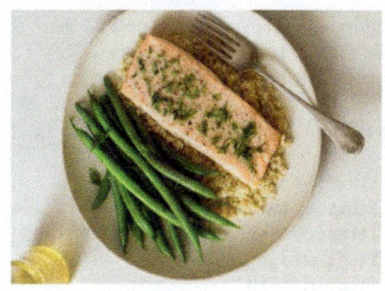

Servings: 2  |  Prep Time: 10 min  |  Cook Time: 15 min  |  Total Time: 25 min
Icons: 🔍 One-Pan  ⏱ Under 30 Min

## Ingredients

- 2 salmon fillets (4 oz each)
- 1 cup cooked quinoa
- 1 cup steamed green beans
- 1 tbsp olive oil
- 1 tsp dried dill
- Juice of 1 lemon

## Directions

1. Heat olive oil in skillet; season salmon with dill and lemon juice.
2. Cook salmon 4–5 minutes per side until flaky.
3. Serve with quinoa and green beans.

**Nutrition (per serving)**

- Calories: 360
- Protein: 34 g
- Carbs: 28 g (Fiber: 6 g)
- Fat: 14 g

**Storage & Prep**

- Refrigerate up to 3 days.
- Salmon freezes separately up to 2 months.

# Spaghetti Squash with Turkey Bolognese

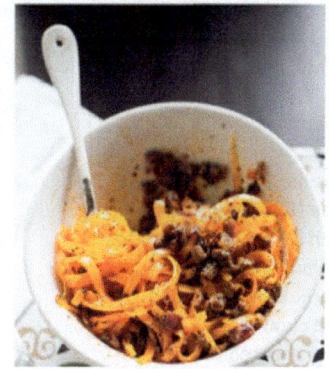

Servings: 4  |  Prep Time: 15 min  |  Cook Time: 40 min  |  Total Time: 55 min
Icons: ❄ Freezer-Friendly  $ Budget-Friendly

## Ingredients

- 1 spaghetti squash, halved and seeded
- 1 lb lean ground turkey
- 1 cup marinara sauce (low sugar)
- 1 onion, diced
- 2 garlic cloves, minced
- 1 tsp Italian seasoning

**Nutrition (per serving)**

- Calories: 320
- Protein: 34 g
- Carbs: 22 g (Fiber: 6 g)
- Fat: 11 g

**Storage & Prep**

- Refrigerate up to 4 days.
- Freeze sauce separately up to 2 months.

## Directions

1. Preheat oven to 400°F (200°C). Roast squash cut-side down for 40 minutes.
2. Meanwhile, brown turkey with onion and garlic. Stir in marinara and Italian seasoning.
3. Scrape squash into strands with fork. Top with turkey sauce.

# Asian Ginger Chicken Lettuce Wraps

Servings: 3 (9 wraps)  |  Prep Time: 10 min  |  Cook
Time: 15 min  |  Total Time: 25 min
Icons: 🔍 One-Pan  ⏱ Under 30 Min

### Ingredients

- 1 lb chicken breast
- 1 tbsp soy sauce
- 1 tbsp hoisin sauce (low sugar if preferred)
- 1 tsp grated ginger
- 1 tsp sesame oil
- 9 large lettuce leaves (romaine or butter)
- ¼ cup shredded carrots

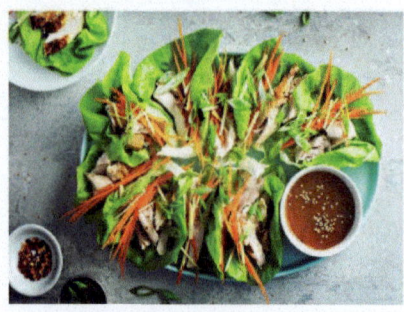

### Directions

1. Heat sesame oil in skillet; cook chicken with ginger until browned. Shred using two forks.
2. Stir in soy sauce and hoisin; simmer 2–3 minutes.
3. Spoon into lettuce leaves and top with shredded carrots.

**Nutrition (per serving = 3 wraps)**

- Calories: 280
- Protein: 30 g
- Carbs: 10 g (Fiber: 3 g)
- Fat: 12 g

**Storage & Prep**

- Refrigerate filling up to 4 days.
- Assemble wraps just before serving.

# Moroccan Chickpea & Chicken Stew

Servings: 4  |  Prep Time: 15 min  |  Cook
Time: 30 min  |  Total Time: 45 min
Icons: 🔍 One-Pan  ❄ Freezer-Friendly

### Ingredients

- 1 lb chicken breast, cubed
- 1 can (15 oz) chickpeas, rinsed
- 1 can (15 oz) diced tomatoes
- 1 onion, diced
- 2 garlic cloves, minced
- 1 tsp cumin
- 1 tsp cinnamon
- 1 tbsp olive oil
- 2 cups chicken broth

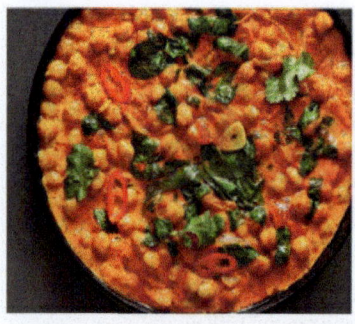

**Nutrition (per serving)**

- Calories: 400
- Protein: 37 g
- Carbs: 32 g (Fiber: 8 g)
- Fat: 13 g

**Storage & Prep**

- Refrigerate up to 5 days.
- Freeze up to 2 months.

### Directions

1. Heat olive oil in pot; cook onion and garlic 3 minutes.
2. Add chicken; cook until browned.
3. Stir in chickpeas, tomatoes, broth, and spices.
4. Simmer 25–30 minutes until stew thickens.

# Mediterranean Baked Chicken Thighs

Servings: 4  |  Prep Time: 10 min  |  Cook
Time: 35 min  |  Total Time: 45 min
Icons: 🔍 One-Pan  ❄️ Freezer-Friendly  $
Budget-Friendly

## Ingredients

- 4 bone-in chicken thighs, skin removed
- 1 tbsp olive oil
- 1 tsp oregano
- 1 tsp paprika
- 1 lemon, sliced
- ½ cup pitted kalamata olives
- 1 cup cherry tomatoes
- Salt & pepper, to taste

## Directions

1. Preheat oven to 400°F (200°C).
2. Rub chicken thighs with olive oil, oregano, paprika, salt, and pepper.
3. Place in baking dish with lemon slices, olives, and tomatoes.
4. Bake 30–35 minutes until internal temp reaches 165°F (74°C).

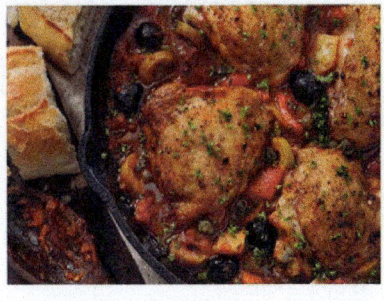

## Nutrition (per serving)

- Calories: 350
- Protein: 36 g
- Carbs: 8 g (Fiber: 2 g)
- Fat: 18 g

## Storage & Prep

- Refrigerate up to 4 days.
- Freeze cooked thighs up to 2 months.

# Chapter 7

# **Plant-Powered Protein**

✦

You don't have to eat meat to hit your protein goals. Plant-based proteins—like beans, lentils, tofu, tempeh, quinoa, edamame, and nuts—pack a powerful punch when combined in smart ways. This chapter proves that high-protein meals can be 100% plant-powered without sacrificing flavor, variety, or satisfaction.

You'll find:

- **Quick weeknight dinners** like tofu stir-fries, lentil curries, and chickpea stews.

- **Hearty salads and bowls** that balance protein, fiber, and healthy fats.

- **Comfort food favorites reimagined** with plant-based swaps that still deliver plenty of protein.

- **Batch-friendly recipes** perfect for meal prep and freezer storage.

Every recipe is designed to provide at least 20–30 grams of protein per serving, using combinations of plant-based staples. Whether you're fully vegan, mostly vegetarian, or just looking to add more plant protein to your week, these dishes will help you feel energized, satisfied, and strong.

# Recipe Icons Guide

🔍 **One-Pan**
Cook the whole meal in a single pan —
less cleanup, more convenience.

❄️ **Freezer-Friendly**
Can be stored in the freezer for later;
reheats well.

💲 **Budget-Friendly**
Costs under $4 per serving with
common ingredients.

⏱️ **Under 30 Minutes**
From prep to plate in half an hour or
less.

⭐ **30+ g Protein**
Each serving delivers at least 30 grams
of protein.

🌱 **Plant-Based**
Fully vegetarian or vegan protein
sources.

# Spicy Lentil & Quinoa Chili

Servings: 4  |  Prep Time: 15 min  |  Cook Time: 30 min  |  Total Time: 45 min
Icons: 🌱 Plant-Based  🍳 One-Pan  ❄️ Freezer-Friendly

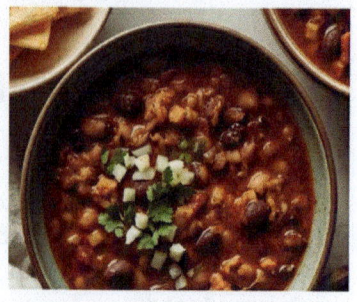

## Ingredients

- 1 cup green or brown lentils, rinsed
- ½ cup quinoa, rinsed
- 1 can (15 oz) black beans, rinsed
- 1 can (15 oz) diced tomatoes
- 1 onion, diced
- 2 garlic cloves, minced
- 1 tbsp chili powder
- 1 tsp cumin
- 4 cups vegetable broth

### Nutrition (per serving)

- Calories: 380
- Protein: 27 g
- Carbs: 62 g (Fiber: 15 g)
- Fat: 6 g

## Directions

1. Heat onion and garlic in pot with splash of oil until softened.
2. Add lentils, quinoa, beans, tomatoes, broth, and spices.
3. Simmer 30 minutes until lentils are tender and chili thickens.

### Storage & Prep

- Refrigerate up to 5 days.
- Freezer-friendly for up to 2 months.

# Teriyaki Tofu & Edamame Bowl

Servings: 2  |  Prep Time: 10 min  |  Cook Time: 15 min  |  Total Time: 25 min
Icons: 🌱 Plant-Based  🍳 One-Pan  ⏱️ Under 30 Min

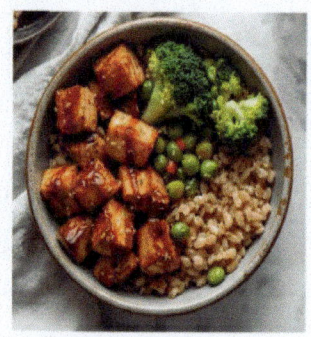

## Ingredients

- 14 oz firm tofu, cubed
- 1 cup shelled edamame
- 1 cup cooked brown rice
- 1 cup broccoli florets
- 2 tbsp teriyaki sauce
- 1 tsp sesame oil

### Nutrition (per serving)

- Calories: 410
- Protein: 32 g
- Carbs: 38 g (Fiber: 9 g)
- Fat: 14 g

## Directions

1. Heat sesame oil in skillet; cook tofu until golden.
2. Stir in teriyaki sauce; cook 2 minutes.
3. Assemble bowls with rice, tofu, edamame, and broccoli.

### Storage & Prep

- Refrigerate up to 4 days.
- Tofu reheats best in skillet.

# Creamy Chickpea & Spinach Curry

Servings: 3 | Prep Time: 10 min | Cook
Time: 20 min | Total Time: 30 min
Icons: 🌱 Plant-Based 🍳 One-Pan ❄️
Freezer-Friendly

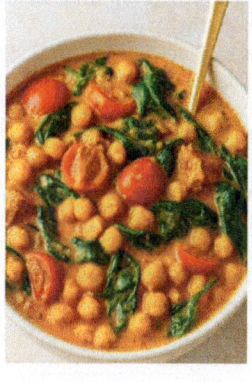

## Ingredients

- 2 cans (15 oz each) chickpeas, rinsed
- 1 onion, diced
- 2 garlic cloves, minced
- 1 cup light coconut milk
- 2 cups spinach
- 1 tbsp curry powder
- 1 tsp cumin
- 1 tbsp olive oil

**Nutrition (per serving)**

- Calories: 360
- Protein: 25 g
- Carbs: 42 g (Fiber: 11 g)
- Fat: 12 g

## Directions

1. Heat oil in pot; cook onion and garlic 3 minutes.
2. Stir in chickpeas, coconut milk, curry powder, and cumin.
3. Simmer 10 minutes, then stir in spinach until wilted.

**Storage & Prep**

- Refrigerate up to 4 days.
- Freeze up to 2 months.

# BBQ Tempeh & Sweet Potato Bowl

Servings: 2 | Prep Time: 10 min | Cook
Time: 20 min | Total Time: 30 min
Icons: 🌱 Plant-Based 🍳 One-Pan $
Budget-Friendly

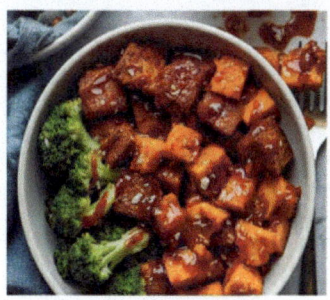

## Ingredients

- 8 oz tempeh, cubed
- 1 medium sweet potato, diced
- 1 cup broccoli florets
- 2 tbsp BBQ sauce (low sugar if preferred)
- 1 tsp olive oil

**Nutrition (per serving)**

- Calories: 370
- Protein: 29 g
- Carbs: 46 g (Fiber: 11 g)
- Fat: 9 g

## Directions

1. Roast sweet potato at 400°F (200°C) for 20 minutes.
2. Heat olive oil in skillet; cook tempeh until golden.
3. Toss tempeh with BBQ sauce.
4. Assemble bowl with sweet potato, broccoli, and tempeh.

**Storage & Prep**

- Refrigerate up to 4 days.
- Tempeh holds texture well for meal prep.

# Mediterranean Lentil Salad

Servings: 4  |  Prep Time: 15 min  |  Total Time: 15 min
Icons: 🌱 Plant-Based  ⏱ Under 30 Min
$ Budget-Friendly

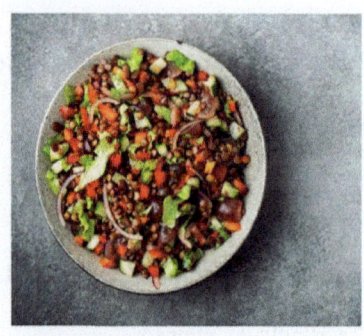

## Ingredients
- 2 cups cooked green lentils
- 1 cup cherry tomatoes, halved
- ½ cucumber, diced
- ¼ red onion, thinly sliced
- ¼ cup kalamata olives, sliced
- 2 tbsp olive oil
- 1 tbsp lemon juice
- 1 tsp oregano

## Directions
1. Combine lentils, tomatoes, cucumber, onion, and olives in bowl.
2. Drizzle with olive oil, lemon juice, and oregano; toss to coat.

### Nutrition (per serving)

- Calories: 310
- Protein: 24 g
- Carbs: 42 g (Fiber: 12 g)
- Fat: 9 g

### Storage & Prep

- Refrigerate up to 4 days.
- Best served chilled.

# Black Bean & Quinoa Stuffed Peppers

Servings: 4  |  Prep Time: 15 min  |  Cook Time: 30 min  |  Total Time: 45 min
Icons: 🌱 Plant-Based  ❄ Freezer-Friendly  $ Budget-Friendly

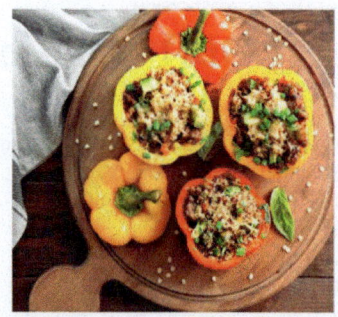

## Ingredients

- 4 large bell peppers, tops removed
- 1 cup cooked quinoa
- 1 can (15 oz) black beans, rinsed
- 1 cup corn kernels
- 1 cup salsa
- 1 tsp cumin

## Directions

1. Preheat oven to 375°F (190°C).
2. Mix quinoa, beans, corn, salsa, and cumin.
3. Stuff peppers with mixture and place in baking dish.
4. Bake 30 minutes until peppers are tender.

### Nutrition (per pepper)

- Calories: 330
- Protein: 23 g
- Carbs: 52 g (Fiber: 11 g)
- Fat: 6 g

### Storage & Prep

- Refrigerate up to 4 days.
- Freeze individually up to 2 months.

# Sesame Ginger Tempeh Stir-Fry

Servings: 2 | Prep Time: 10 min | Cook Time: 15 min | Total Time: 25 min
Icons: 🌱 Plant-Based 🍳 One-Pan ⏱ Under 30 Min

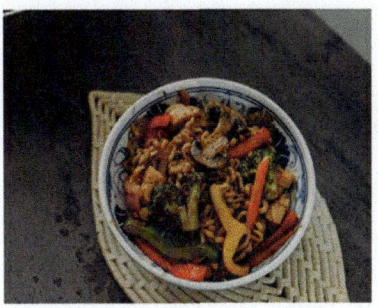

## Ingredients

- 8 oz tempeh, cubed
- 2 cups mixed stir-fry vegetables
- 2 tbsp soy sauce
- 1 tbsp rice vinegar
- 1 tsp sesame oil
- 1 tsp grated ginger

## Directions

1. Heat sesame oil in skillet; cook tempeh until golden.
2. Add vegetables, soy sauce, vinegar, and ginger; stir-fry 6–7 minutes.
3. Serve hot.

## Nutrition (per serving)

- Calories: 350
- Protein: 29 g
- Carbs: 28 g (Fiber: 8 g)
- Fat: 14 g

## Storage & Prep

- Refrigerate up to 4 days.
- Best reheated in skillet to keep texture.

# High-Protein Vegan Shepherd's Pie

Servings: 4 | Prep Time: 20 min | Cook Time: 25 min | Total Time: 45 min
Icons: 🌱 Plant-Based ❄ Freezer-Friendly

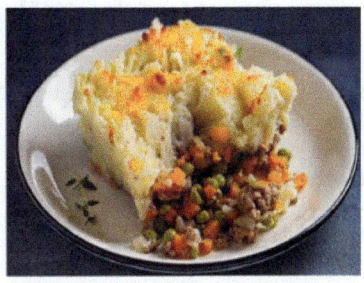

## Ingredients

- 1 cup cooked lentils
- 1 cup frozen peas and carrots
- 1 onion, diced
- 1 cup vegetable broth
- 1 tbsp tomato paste
- 1 tsp thyme
- 2 cups mashed potatoes (made with plant milk)

## Nutrition (per serving)

- Calories: 390
- Protein: 25 g
- Carbs: 56 g (Fiber: 12 g)
- Fat: 10 g

## Directions

1. Preheat oven to 375°F (190°C).
2. Heat onion in skillet; add lentils, peas, carrots, broth, tomato paste, and thyme. Simmer 10 minutes.
3. Spread mixture in baking dish; top with mashed potatoes.
4. Bake 20–25 minutes until golden on top.

## Storage & Prep

- Refrigerate up to 4 days.
- Freezer-friendly up to 2 months.

# Peanut Tofu Power Bowl

Servings: 2  |  Prep Time: 10 min  |  Cook Time: 15 min  |  Total Time: 25 min
Icons: 🌱 Plant-Based  🍳 One-Pan  ⏱ Under 30 Min

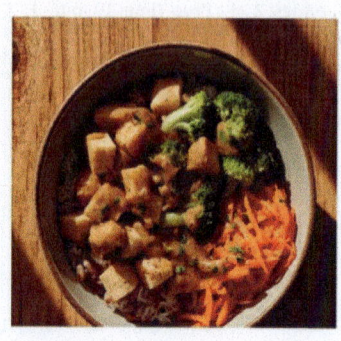

## Ingredients

- 14 oz firm tofu, cubed
- 1 cup cooked brown rice
- 1 cup steamed broccoli
- 1 carrot, shredded
- 2 tbsp peanut butter
- 1 tbsp soy sauce
- 1 tsp sriracha

## Directions

1. Pan-fry tofu until golden.
2. In small bowl, whisk peanut butter, soy sauce, and sriracha with splash of water.
3. Assemble bowls with rice, broccoli, carrot, tofu, and drizzle peanut sauce on top.

### Nutrition (per serving)

- Calories: 420
- Protein: 31 g
- Carbs: 38 g (Fiber: 8 g)
- Fat: 17 g

### Storage & Prep

- Refrigerate up to 4 days.
- Sauce stores separately up to 1 week.

# Red Lentil & Spinach Dhal

Servings: 4  |  Prep Time: 10 min  |  Cook Time: 25 min  |  Total Time: 35 min
Icons: 🌱 Plant-Based  🍳 One-Pan  ❄️ Freezer-Friendly

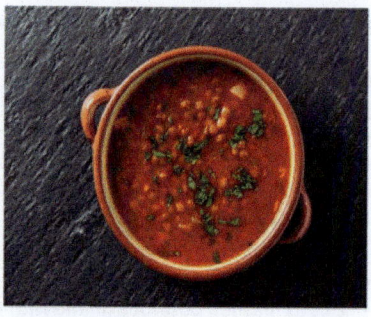

## Ingredients

- 1 cup red lentils, rinsed
- 4 cups vegetable broth
- 1 onion, diced
- 2 garlic cloves, minced
- 1 tsp turmeric
- 1 tsp cumin
- 2 cups spinach
- 1 tbsp olive oil

## Directions

1. Heat oil in pot; cook onion and garlic 3 minutes.
2. Add lentils, broth, turmeric, and cumin; simmer 20–25 minutes until creamy.
3. Stir in spinach until wilted.

### Nutrition (per serving)

- Calories: 330
- Protein: 26 g
- Carbs: 47 g (Fiber: 14 g)
- Fat: 7 g

### Storage & Prep

- Refrigerate up to 5 days.
- Freeze up to 2 months.

# Chickpea & Avocado Wraps

Servings: 2  |  Prep Time: 10 min  |  Total Time: 10 min

Icons: 🌱 Plant-Based  ⏲ Under 30 Min  $ Budget-Friendly

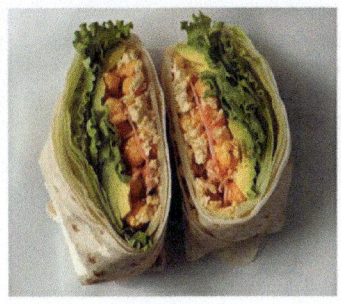

## Ingredients

- 1 can (15 oz) chickpeas, rinsed and mashed
- 1 avocado, mashed
- 1 tbsp lemon juice
- 1 tsp garlic powder
- 4 whole wheat tortillas
- 1 cup shredded lettuce

**Nutrition (per wrap)**

- Calories: 290
- Protein: 22 g
- Carbs: 38 g (Fiber: 10 g)
- Fat: 9 g

## Directions

1. Mix chickpeas, avocado, lemon juice, and garlic powder.
2. Spread mixture onto tortillas, top with lettuce, and roll up.

**Storage & Prep**

- Best enjoyed fresh.
- Filling can be refrigerated up to 2 days.

# Smoky Black Bean Burgers

Servings: 4  |  Prep Time: 15 min  |  Cook Time: 15 min  |  Total Time: 30 min

Icons: 🌱 Plant-Based  🔍 One-Pan  ❄ Freezer-Friendly

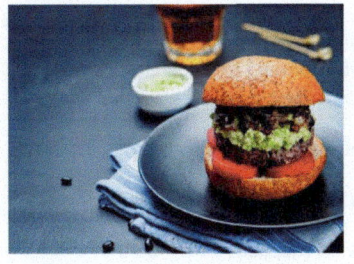

## Ingredients

- 2 cans (15 oz each) black beans, rinsed and mashed
- ½ cup breadcrumbs (GF option: oat flour)
- ¼ cup onion, diced
- 1 tsp smoked paprika
- 1 tsp cumin
- 2 tbsp olive oil

**Nutrition (per patty)**

- Calories: 250
- Protein: 20 g
- Carbs: 34 g (Fiber: 10 g)
- Fat: 7 g

## Directions

1. Mix beans, breadcrumbs, onion, paprika, and cumin into patties.
2. Heat oil in skillet; cook patties 4–5 minutes per side.

**Storage & Prep**

- Refrigerate up to 4 days.
- Freeze patties uncooked up to 2 months.

# Vegan Pad Thai with Tofu

Servings: 3  |  Prep Time: 15 min  |  Cook Time: 15 min  |  Total Time: 30 min
Icons: 🌱 Plant-Based  🔍 One-Pan  🕐 Under 30 Min

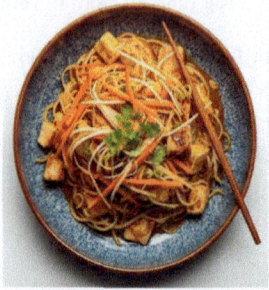

## Ingredients

- 8 oz rice noodles
- 14 oz firm tofu, cubed
- 1 cup bean sprouts
- 1 carrot, shredded
- 2 tbsp soy sauce
- 1 tbsp peanut butter
- 1 tbsp lime juice
- 1 tsp chili paste (optional)

### Nutrition (per serving)

- Calories: 410
- Protein: 29 g
- Carbs: 54 g (Fiber: 7 g)
- Fat: 11 g

## Directions

1. Cook noodles per package instructions.
2. Pan-fry tofu until golden.
3. Toss noodles, tofu, sprouts, carrot, soy sauce, peanut butter, lime juice, and chili paste.

### Storage & Prep

- Refrigerate up to 3 days.
- Best reheated in skillet with splash of water.

# White Bean & Kale Stew

Servings: 4  |  Prep Time: 10 min  |  Cook Time: 25 min  |  Total Time: 35 min
Icons: 🌱 Plant-Based  🔍 One-Pan  ❄️ Freezer-Friendly

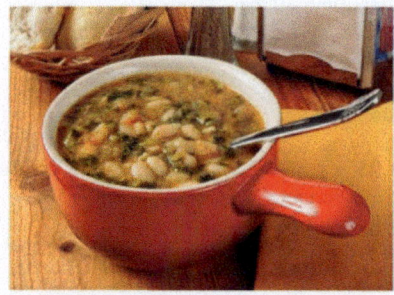

## Ingredients

- 2 cans (15 oz each) white beans, rinsed
- 4 cups vegetable broth
- 2 cups kale, chopped
- 1 onion, diced
- 2 garlic cloves, minced
- 1 tsp thyme
- 1 tbsp olive oil

### Nutrition (per serving)

- Calories: 330
- Protein: 24 g
- Carbs: 46 g (Fiber: 12 g)
- Fat: 8 g

## Directions

1. Heat oil in pot; cook onion and garlic until soft.
2. Add beans, broth, and thyme; simmer 15 minutes.
3. Stir in kale and cook 5 minutes until tender.

### Storage & Prep

- Refrigerate up to 4 days.
- Freeze up to 2 months.

# Mediterranean Hummus Bowl

Servings: 2  |  Prep Time: 10 min  |  Total Time: 10 min
Icons: 🌱 Plant-Based  ⏱ Under 30 Min

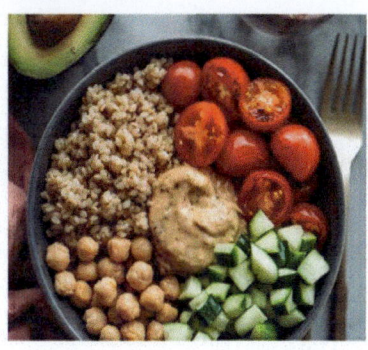

## Ingredients

- 1 cup hummus
- 1 cup cooked farro or quinoa
- 1 cup roasted chickpeas
- 1 cup cherry tomatoes, halved
- ½ cucumber, diced
- 2 tbsp olive oil
- 1 tsp oregano

## Directions

1. Assemble bowls with hummus, farro, chickpeas, tomatoes, and cucumber.
2. Drizzle with olive oil and sprinkle with oregano.

Nutrition (per serving)

- Calories: 380
- Protein: 27 g
- Carbs: 48 g (Fiber: 11 g)
- Fat: 12 g

Storage & Prep

- Refrigerate up to 3 days.
- Best served chilled.

# Curried Red Lentil Soup

Servings: 4  |  Prep Time: 10 min  |  Cook Time: 25 min  |  Total Time: 35 min
Icons: 🌱 Plant-Based  🍳 One-Pan  ❄️ Freezer-Friendly

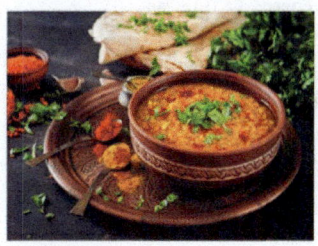

## Ingredients

- 1 cup red lentils, rinsed
- 4 cups vegetable broth
- 1 can (15 oz) diced tomatoes
- 1 onion, diced
- 2 garlic cloves, minced
- 1 tbsp curry powder
- 1 tsp turmeric
- 1 tbsp olive oil

## Directions

1. Heat olive oil in pot; sauté onion and garlic until softened.
2. Stir in curry powder and turmeric.
3. Add lentils, broth, and tomatoes. Simmer 20–25 minutes until creamy.

Nutrition (per serving)

- Calories: 330
- Protein: 26 g
- Carbs: 47 g (Fiber: 12 g)
- Fat: 7 g

Storage & Prep

- Refrigerate up to 5 days.
- Freeze up to 2 months.

# Tofu & Vegetable Fried "Rice" (Cauliflower Base)

Servings: 3  |  Prep Time: 10 min  |  Cook Time: 15 min  |  Total Time: 25 min
Icons: 🌱 Plant-Based  🍳 One-Pan  ⏲ Under 30 Min

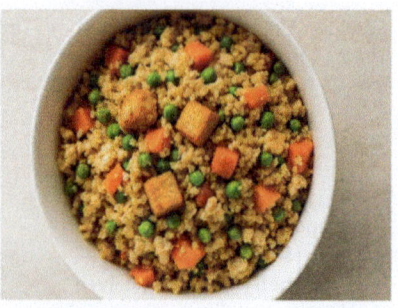

### Ingredients

- 14 oz firm tofu, cubed
- 3 cups riced cauliflower
- 1 cup mixed frozen vegetables (peas, corn, carrots)
- 2 tbsp soy sauce
- 1 tsp sesame oil
- 1 tsp grated ginger

### Nutrition (per serving)

- Calories: 290
- Protein: 24 g
- Carbs: 22 g (Fiber: 7 g)
- Fat: 12 g

### Directions

1. Heat sesame oil in skillet; cook tofu until golden.
2. Add cauliflower rice, vegetables, soy sauce, and ginger.
3. Stir-fry 6–7 minutes until heated through.

### Storage & Prep

- Refrigerate up to 4 days.
- Best reheated in skillet, not microwave.

# Vegan Mushroom Stroganoff

Servings: 4  |  Prep Time: 15 min  |  Cook Time: 20 min  |  Total Time: 35 min
Icons: 🌱 Plant-Based  🍳 One-Pan  ❄ Freezer-Friendly

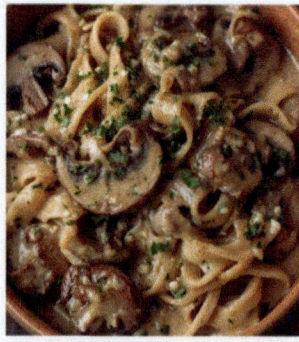

### Ingredients

- 12 oz mushrooms, sliced
- 1 onion, diced
- 2 garlic cloves, minced
- 1 cup cashew cream (blend soaked cashews + water)
- 1 cup vegetable broth
- 1 tsp paprika
- 8 oz whole wheat pasta

### Nutrition (per serving)

- Calories: 410
- Protein: 25 g
- Carbs: 56 g (Fiber: 9 g)
- Fat: 12 g

### Directions

1. Cook pasta according to package instructions.
2. Heat skillet; sauté onion, garlic, and mushrooms until soft.
3. Stir in broth, cashew cream, and paprika; simmer 5 minutes.
4. Toss sauce with pasta.

### Storage & Prep

- Refrigerate up to 4 days.
- Freeze sauce separately for up to 2 months.

# Edamame & Brown Rice Power Bowl

Servings: 2  |  Prep Time: 10 min  |  Total Time: 10 min
Icons: 🌱 Plant-Based   ⏱ Under 30 Min
💲 Budget-Friendly

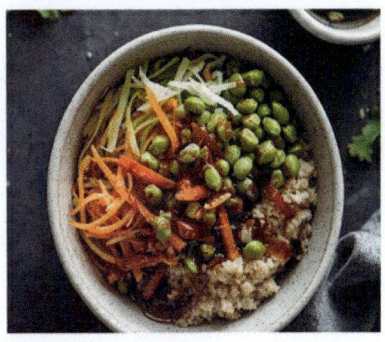

## Ingredients

- 2 cups cooked brown rice
- 1 cup shelled edamame
- 1 cup shredded cabbage
- 1 carrot, shredded
- 2 tbsp soy sauce
- 1 tsp sesame oil

## Directions

1. Divide rice between two bowls.
2. Top with edamame, cabbage, and carrot.
3. Drizzle with soy sauce and sesame oil.

### Nutrition (per serving)

- Calories: 350
- Protein: 28 g
- Carbs: 48 g (Fiber: 10 g)
- Fat: 9 g

### Storage & Prep

- Refrigerate up to 4 days.
- Best enjoyed cold or room temperature.

# Vegan Protein Pasta Primavera

Servings: 4  |  Prep Time: 10 min  |  Cook Time: 15 min  |  Total Time: 25 min
Icons: 🌱 Plant-Based   🔍 One-Pan   ⏱ Under 30 Min

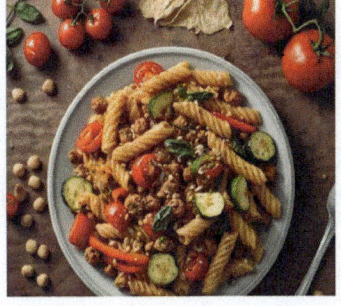

## Ingredients

- 12 oz chickpea or lentil pasta
- 1 cup zucchini, sliced
- 1 cup bell peppers, sliced
- 1 cup cherry tomatoes, halved
- 2 garlic cloves, minced
- 1 tbsp olive oil
- 1 tsp Italian seasoning

## Directions

1. Cook pasta according to package instructions.
2. Heat olive oil; sauté garlic and vegetables until softened.
3. Toss with pasta and Italian seasoning.

### Nutrition (per serving)

- Calories: 400
- Protein: 29 g
- Carbs: 56 g (Fiber: 12 g)
- Fat: 9 g

### Storage & Prep

- Refrigerate up to 4 days.
- Best reheated in skillet with splash of water.

# Vegan Sloppy Joes (Lentil-Based)

Servings: 4 | Prep Time: 10 min | Cook Time: 20 min | Total Time: 30 min
Icons: 🌱 Plant-Based 🍳 One-Pan ❄️ Freezer-Friendly

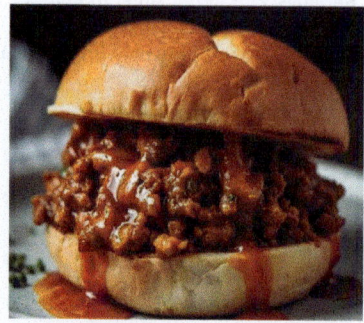

## Ingredients

- 1 cup cooked lentils
- 1 cup tomato sauce
- 1 tbsp tomato paste
- 1 onion, diced
- 1 tbsp soy sauce
- 1 tsp smoked paprika
- 4 whole wheat buns

## Directions

1. Heat skillet; cook onion until soft.
2. Stir in lentils, tomato sauce, tomato paste, soy sauce, and paprika.
3. Simmer 10–15 minutes until thick.
4. Serve on buns.

### Nutrition (per serving)

- Calories: 360
- Protein: 26 g
- Carbs: 54 g (Fiber: 10 g)
- Fat: 7 g

### Storage & Prep

- Refrigerate up to 4 days.
- Freeze filling separately up to 2 months.

# Vegan Chickpea "Chicken" Salad

Servings: 3 | Prep Time: 10 min | Total Time: 10 min
Icons: 🌱 Plant-Based ⏱ Under 30 Min $ Budget-Friendly

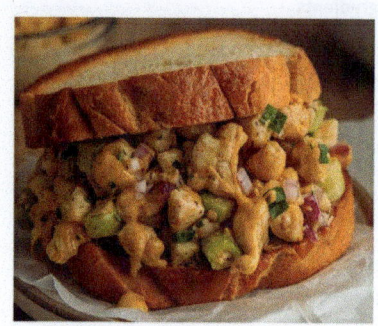

## Ingredients

- 2 cans (15 oz each) chickpeas, rinsed and mashed
- ¼ cup vegan mayo (or mashed avocado)
- 1 celery stalk, diced
- 2 tbsp red onion, diced
- 1 tsp Dijon mustard
- Salt & pepper, to taste

## Directions

1. Mix chickpeas, mayo, celery, onion, mustard, salt, and pepper.
2. Serve as sandwich filling or over greens.

### Nutrition (per serving)

- Calories: 300
- Protein: 23 g
- Carbs: 38 g (Fiber: 9 g)
- Fat: 9 g

### Storage & Prep

- Refrigerate up to 3 days.
- Not freezer-friendly.

# Sweet Potato & Black Bean Enchiladas

Servings: 4 | Prep Time: 20 min | Cook Time: 25 min | Total Time: 45 min
Icons: 🌱 Plant-Based ❄️ Freezer-Friendly

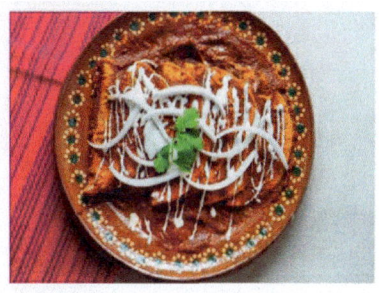

## Ingredients

- 2 medium sweet potatoes, diced and roasted
- 1 can (15 oz) black beans, rinsed
- 1 cup enchilada sauce
- 8 small whole wheat tortillas
- ½ cup dairy-free shredded cheese (optional)

## Directions

1. Preheat oven to 375°F (190°C).
2. Mash roasted sweet potato and mix with black beans.
3. Roll into tortillas, place in baking dish, and cover with enchilada sauce.
4. Sprinkle cheese if using. Bake 20–25 minutes.

**Nutrition (per serving = 2 enchiladas)**

- Calories: 390
- Protein: 27 g
- Carbs: 60 g (Fiber: 13 g)
- Fat: 9 g

**Storage & Prep**

- Refrigerate up to 4 days.
- Freeze assembled enchiladas up to 2 months.

# Tempeh Tacos with Avocado Crema

Servings: 3 (6 tacos) | Prep Time: 10 min | Cook Time: 10 min | Total Time: 20 min
Icons: 🌱 Plant-Based 🔍 One-Pan ⏱️ Under 30 Min

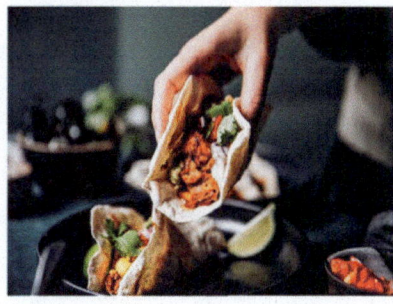

## Ingredients

- 8 oz tempeh, crumbled
- 1 tbsp soy sauce
- 1 tsp chili powder
- 1 tsp cumin
- 6 corn tortillas
- 1 avocado
- 2 tbsp lime juice
- 2 tbsp dairy-free yogurt

**Nutrition (per serving = 2 tacos)**

- Calories: 340
- Protein: 28 g
- Carbs: 32 g (Fiber: 9 g)
- Fat: 12 g

## Directions

1. Cook tempeh with soy sauce, chili powder, and cumin in skillet until golden.
2. Mash avocado with lime juice and yogurt for crema.
3. Fill tortillas with tempeh and drizzle with crema.

**Storage & Prep**

- Refrigerate filling up to 4 days.
- Assemble tacos just before serving.

# Chapter 8

# High-Protein Snacks & Small Bites

✦

Snacking doesn't have to mean empty calories or blood sugar crashes. With the right ingredients, your between-meal bites can be just as powerful as your main meals—helping you stay energized, curb cravings, and hit your protein goals without effort.

In this chapter, you'll find more than 15 snack recipes that deliver a satisfying punch of protein in every bite. From portable grab-and-go options like protein muffins and energy balls, to savory favorites like roasted chickpeas and veggie dips, to sweet but smart treats like yogurt parfaits and no-bake bars—you'll always have a quick, nourishing choice at hand.

Each recipe is designed to be easy, prep-friendly, and portion-controlled so you can fuel your day without derailing your goals. Whether you need a post-workout boost, a mid-afternoon tide-me-over, or a late-night bite that won't wreck your progress, these small but mighty snacks have you covered.

# Recipe Icons Guide

🔍 **One-Pan**
Cook the whole meal in a single pan —
less cleanup, more convenience.

❄️ **Freezer-Friendly**
Can be stored in the freezer for later;
reheats well.

$ **Budget-Friendly**
Costs under $4 per serving with
common ingredients.

🕐 **Under 30 Minutes**
From prep to plate in half an hour or
less.

⭐ **30+ g Protein**
Each serving delivers at least 30 grams
of protein.

🌱 **Plant-Based**
Fully vegetarian or vegan protein
sources.

# Roasted Chickpeas Crunch

Servings: 4  |  Prep Time: 5 min  |  Cook Time: 30 min  |  Total Time: 35 min
Icons: 🌱 Plant-Based  🕐 Under 30 Min  $ Budget-Friendly

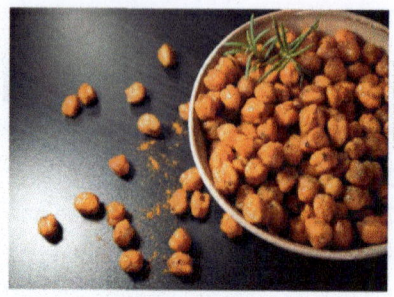

## Ingredients

- 2 cans (15 oz each) chickpeas, rinsed and dried
- 1 tbsp olive oil
- 1 tsp smoked paprika
- ½ tsp garlic powder
- ½ tsp salt

## Directions

1. Preheat oven to 400°F (200°C).
2. Toss chickpeas with olive oil and seasonings.
3. Spread on baking sheet; roast 25–30 minutes until crisp.

### Nutrition (per serving)

- Calories: 210
- Protein: 14 g
- Carbs: 28 g (Fiber: 7 g)
- Fat: 6 g

### Storage & Prep

- Store in airtight container up to 5 days.
- Best enjoyed at room temperature.

# Cottage Cheese Berry Parfait

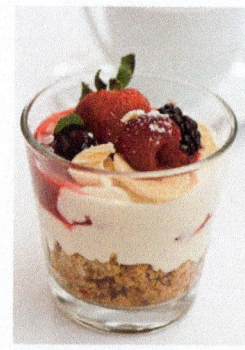

Servings: 2  |  Prep Time: 5 min  |  Total Time: 5 min
Icons: 🕐 Under 30 Min  $ Budget-Friendly

## Ingredients

- 1 cup low-fat cottage cheese
- 1 cup mixed berries (blueberries, strawberries, raspberries)
- 2 tbsp granola
- 1 tsp honey (optional)

## Directions

1. Layer cottage cheese, berries, and granola in cups.
2. Drizzle with honey if desired.

### Nutrition (per serving)

- Calories: 220
- Protein: 21 g
- Carbs: 26 g (Fiber: 4 g)
- Fat: 4 g

### Storage & Prep

- Assemble just before serving.
- Store components separately up to 3 days.

# High-Protein Hummus Dip

Servings: 6  |  Prep Time: 10 min  |  Total Time: 10 min
Icons: 🌱 Plant-Based   ⏱ Under 30 Min
$ Budget-Friendly

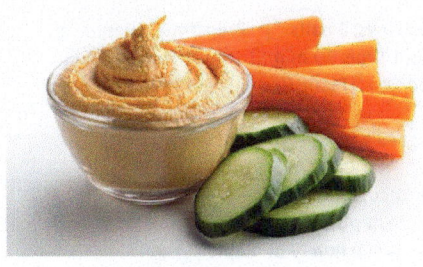

## Ingredients

- 2 cans (15 oz each) chickpeas, rinsed
- 3 tbsp tahini
- Juice of 1 lemon
- 2 garlic cloves
- 1 tsp cumin
- ¼ cup water (adjust for texture)

## Directions

1. Blend all ingredients until smooth.
2. Adjust consistency with water.

**Nutrition (per serving, ¼ cup)**

- Calories: 160
- Protein: 12 g
- Carbs: 18 g (Fiber: 5 g)
- Fat: 5 g

**Storage & Prep**

- Refrigerate up to 5 days.
- Freeze in portions up to 2 months.

# Turkey & Cheese Roll-Ups

Servings: 2  |  Prep Time: 5 min  |  Total Time: 5 min
Icons: ⏱ Under 30 Min   $ Budget-Friendly

## Ingredients

- 6 slices deli turkey (low sodium)
- 3 slices cheese (cheddar or Swiss), halved
- 6 cucumber sticks

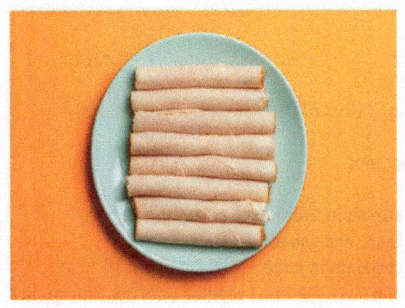

## Directions

1. Layer turkey with cheese and cucumber stick.
2. Roll up and secure with toothpick.

**Nutrition (per serving)**

- Calories: 200
- Protein: 25 g
- Carbs: 3 g (Fiber: 1 g)
- Fat: 10 g

**Storage & Prep**

- Best eaten fresh.
- Can refrigerate up to 2 days.

# Chocolate Peanut Butter Protein Balls

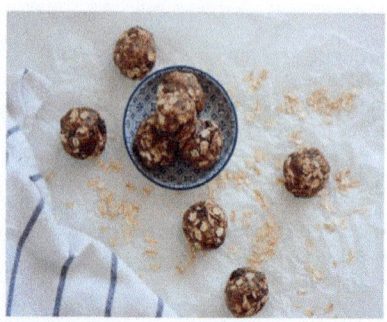

Servings: 8 balls | Prep Time: 10 min |
Chill Time: 30 min | Total Time: 40 min
Icons: 🌱 Plant-Based ❄️ Freezer-Friendly

## Ingredients

- 1 cup rolled oats
- ½ cup peanut butter
- ¼ cup honey or maple syrup
- ¼ cup chocolate protein powder
- 2 tbsp cocoa powder

## Directions

1. Mix all ingredients until combined.
2. Roll into balls; chill 30 minutes before serving.

**Nutrition (per ball)**

- Calories: 140
- Protein: 8 g
- Carbs: 15 g (Fiber: 3 g)
- Fat: 6 g

**Storage & Prep**

- Refrigerate up to 1 week.
- Freeze up to 2 months.

# Greek Yogurt Ranch Dip with Veggies

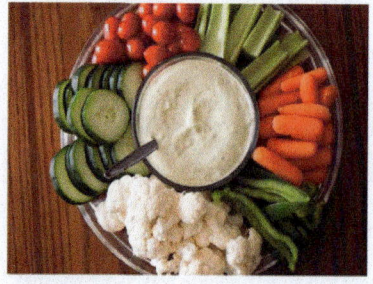

Servings: 4 | Prep Time: 5 min | Total Time: 5 min
Icons: 🕐 Under 30 Min   $ Budget-Friendly

## Ingredients

- 1 cup plain Greek yogurt (2% or fat-free)
- 1 tbsp ranch seasoning mix
- 1 tbsp lemon juice
- 2 cups assorted raw veggies (carrots, celery, bell peppers)

## Directions

1. Stir yogurt, ranch seasoning, and lemon juice until smooth.
2. Serve with raw veggies for dipping.

**Nutrition (per serving, dip only)**

- Calories: 120
- Protein: 14 g
- Carbs: 8 g (Fiber: 2 g)
- Fat: 3 g

**Storage & Prep**

- Refrigerate dip up to 4 days.
- Store veggies separately for crispness.

# Edamame with Sea Salt

Servings: 2  |  Prep Time: 5 min  |  Cook Time: 5 min  |  Total Time: 10 min
Icons: 🌱 Plant-Based  🕙 Under 30 Min  $ Budget-Friendly

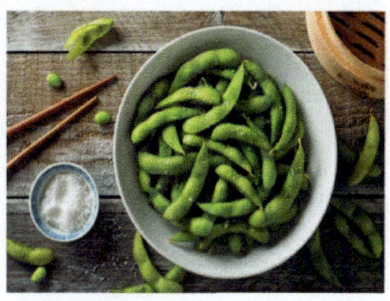

## Ingredients

- 2 cups frozen edamame in pods
- 1 tsp sea salt
- ½ tsp sesame seeds (optional)

## Directions

1. Boil or steam edamame 5 minutes. Drain.
2. Sprinkle with sea salt and sesame seeds if desired.

## Nutrition (per serving)

- Calories: 190
- Protein: 18 g
- Carbs: 16 g (Fiber: 5 g)
- Fat: 7 g

## Storage & Prep

- Best eaten fresh.
- Refrigerate leftovers up to 2 days.

# Protein-Packed Deviled Eggs

Servings: 4 (8 halves)  |  Prep Time: 10 min  |  Total Time: 10 min
Icons: 🕙 Under 30 Min  $ Budget-Friendly

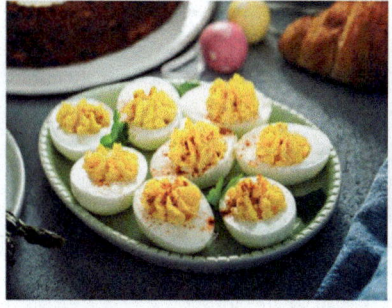

## Ingredients

- 4 hard-boiled eggs, halved
- 2 tbsp Greek yogurt
- 1 tsp Dijon mustard
- ½ tsp paprika
- Salt & pepper, to taste

## Directions

1. Remove yolks and mash with yogurt, mustard, salt, and pepper.
2. Spoon mixture back into egg whites. Sprinkle with paprika.

## Nutrition (per 2 halves)

- Calories: 120
- Protein: 12 g
- Carbs: 2 g (Fiber: 0 g)
- Fat: 7 g

## Storage & Prep

- Refrigerate up to 3 days.
- Not freezer-friendly.

# Almond Butter Apple Slices

Servings: 2  |  Prep Time: 5 min  |  Total Time: 5 min
Icons: 🌱 Plant-Based  ⏱ Under 30 Min

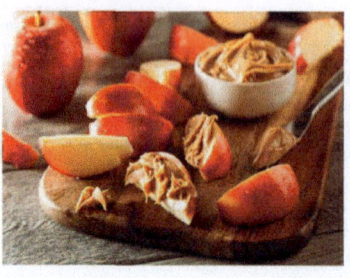

### Ingredients

- 2 medium apples, sliced
- 4 tbsp almond butter
- 1 tbsp chia seeds (optional topping)

### Directions

1. Slice apples and spread with almond butter.
2. Sprinkle with chia seeds if desired.

**Nutrition (per serving)**

- Calories: 260
- Protein: 9 g
- Carbs: 34 g (Fiber: 7 g)
- Fat: 12 g

**Storage & Prep**

- Best eaten fresh.
- Apples brown quickly; drizzle with lemon juice if storing.

# No-Bake Protein Brownie Bites

Servings: 8 bites  |  Prep Time: 10 min  |
Chill Time: 30 min  |  Total Time: 40 min
Icons: 🌱 Plant-Based  ❄ Freezer-Friendly

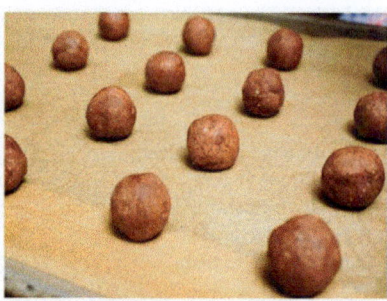

### Ingredients

- 1 cup dates, pitted
- ½ cup almond flour
- ¼ cup chocolate protein powder
- 2 tbsp cocoa powder
- 2 tbsp almond butter

### Directions

1. Blend all ingredients until dough forms.
2. Roll into balls and chill 30 minutes.

**Nutrition (per bite)**

- Calories: 120
- Protein: 7 g
- Carbs: 16 g (Fiber: 3 g)
- Fat: 6 g

**Storage & Prep**

- Refrigerate up to 1 week.
- Freeze up to 2 months.

# Tuna & Avocado Stuffed Cucumbers

Servings: 2  |  Prep Time: 10 min  |  Total Time: 10 min
Icons: ⏱ Under 30 Min   $ Budget-Friendly

## Ingredients

- 1 can (5 oz) tuna, drained
- ½ avocado, mashed
- 1 tbsp Greek yogurt
- 1 cucumber, cut into thick slices and hollowed slightly
- ½ tsp lemon juice

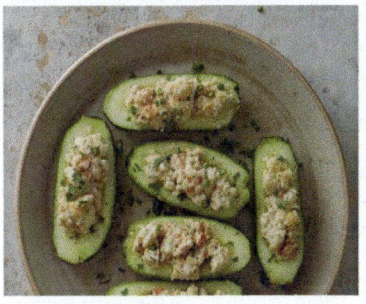

## Directions

1. Mix tuna, avocado, yogurt, and lemon juice.
2. Spoon mixture into cucumber slices.

### Nutrition (per serving)

- Calories: 210
- Protein: 22 g
- Carbs: 9 g (Fiber: 3 g)
- Fat: 10 g

### Storage & Prep

- Best eaten fresh.
- Filling can be prepped up to 2 days in advance.

# Spicy Roasted Edamame

Servings: 4  |  Prep Time: 5 min  |  Cook Time: 20 min  |  Total Time: 25 min
Icons: 🌱 Plant-Based   ⏱ Under 30 Min   $ Budget-Friendly

## Ingredients

- 3 cups shelled edamame
- 1 tbsp olive oil
- 1 tsp chili powder
- ½ tsp garlic powder
- ½ tsp sea salt

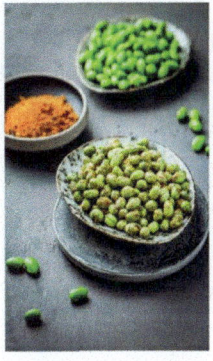

## Directions

1. Preheat oven to 400°F (200°C).
2. Toss edamame with olive oil and seasonings.
3. Spread on baking sheet; roast 20 minutes until crisp.

### Nutrition (per serving)

- Calories: 180
- Protein: 19 g
- Carbs: 15 g (Fiber: 5 g)
- Fat: 6 g

### Storage & Prep

- Store in airtight container up to 4 days.
- Best enjoyed warm.

# High-Protein Trail Mix

Servings: 6  |  Prep Time: 5 min  |  Total Time: 5 min
Icons: 🌱 Plant-Based  🕐 Under 30 Min  ❄️ Freezer-Friendly

### Ingredients

- 1 cup roasted almonds
- 1 cup roasted chickpeas
- ½ cup pumpkin seeds
- ½ cup dried cranberries
- ½ cup dark chocolate chips

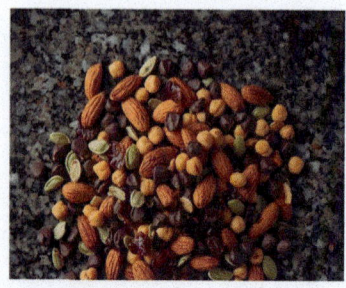

### Directions

1. Mix all ingredients in large bowl.
2. Portion into snack bags for easy grab-and-go.

**Nutrition (per serving)**

- Calories: 240
- Protein: 12 g
- Carbs: 22 g (Fiber: 5 g)
- Fat: 12 g

**Storage & Prep**

- Store in airtight container up to 2 weeks.
- Freeze up to 2 months.

# Mini Egg Muffins

Servings: 4 (8 muffins)  |  Prep Time: 10 min  |  Cook Time: 20 min  |  Total Time: 30 min
Icons: 🕐 Under 30 Min  ❄️ Freezer-Friendly

### Ingredients

- 6 eggs
- ½ cup diced bell peppers
- ½ cup spinach, chopped
- ¼ cup shredded cheddar
- Salt & pepper, to taste

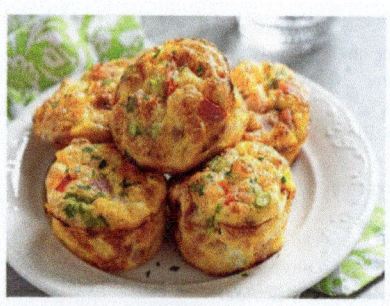

**Nutrition (per 2 muffins)**

- Calories: 160
- Protein: 14 g
- Carbs: 4 g (Fiber: 1 g)
- Fat: 9 g

### Directions

1. Preheat oven to 375°F (190°C). Grease muffin tin.
2. Whisk eggs with salt and pepper. Stir in peppers, spinach, and cheese.
3. Pour into muffin cups and bake 18–20 minutes until set.

**Storage & Prep**

- Refrigerate up to 4 days.
- Freeze up to 2 months.

# Protein-Packed Chia Pudding

Servings: 2 | Prep Time: 5 min | Chill
Time: 4 hrs | Total Time: 4 hrs+
Icons: 🌱 Plant-Based ❄️ Freezer-Friendly

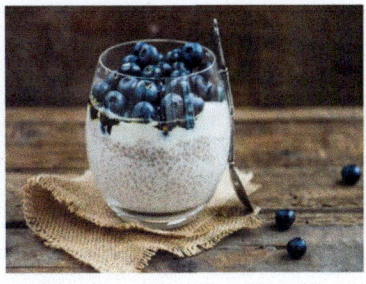

## Ingredients

- ½ cup chia seeds
- 2 cups unsweetened almond milk
- 1 scoop vanilla protein powder
- 1 tsp maple syrup (optional)
- ½ cup berries (for topping)

## Directions

1. Mix chia seeds, almond milk, protein powder, and maple syrup.
2. Stir well; refrigerate 4 hours or overnight until thick.
3. Top with berries before serving.

### Nutrition (per serving)

- Calories: 280
- Protein: 23 g
- Carbs: 24 g (Fiber: 9 g)
- Fat: 10 g

### Storage & Prep

- Refrigerate up to 5 days.
- Freeze in single-serve jars up to 1 month.

# Chapter 9

# Sweets & Treats

✦

Yes—you can satisfy your sweet tooth and still stay on track with your high-protein goals. Desserts don't have to mean empty calories or guilt. With a few smart swaps and protein-rich ingredients, you can enjoy cookies, brownies, puddings, and frozen treats that fuel your body as well as your cravings.

In this chapter, you'll find more than 10 recipes that are easy to make, prep-friendly, and family-approved. From no-bake bars and protein cookies to chocolate classics reimagined with protein powder, these treats strike the balance between indulgent and nourishing.

Each recipe is built to deliver satisfying sweetness with 10–20 grams of protein per serving, so you can feel good about dessert time—whether it's post-workout, after dinner, or as a mid-afternoon pick-me-up.

# Recipe Icons Guide

🔍 **One-Pan**
Cook the whole meal in a single pan — less cleanup, more convenience.

❄️ **Freezer-Friendly**
Can be stored in the freezer for later; reheats well.

$ **Budget-Friendly**
Costs under $4 per serving with common ingredients.

⏱ **Under 30 Minutes**
From prep to plate in half an hour or less.

⭐ **30+ g Protein**
Each serving delivers at least 30 grams of protein.

🌱 **Plant-Based**
Fully vegetarian or vegan protein sources.

# High-Protein Cheesecake Bites

Servings: 8 bites | Prep Time: 15 min | Chill Time: 2 hrs | Total Time: 2 hrs 15 min
Icons: ❄ Freezer-Friendly ⏱ Under 30 Min

### Ingredients

- 1 cup low-fat cream cheese
- ½ cup Greek yogurt
- ½ cup vanilla protein powder
- 2 tbsp honey or maple syrup
- ½ cup crushed graham crackers (or almond flour for GF)

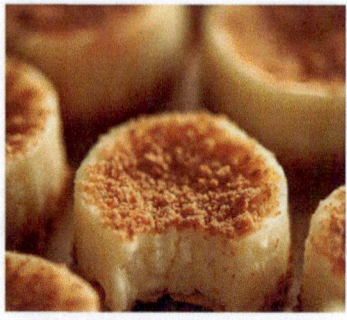

### Directions

1. Mix cream cheese, yogurt, protein powder, and honey until smooth.
2. Scoop into bite-sized silicone molds.
3. Sprinkle with graham crumbs.
4. Chill at least 2 hours until set.

Nutrition (per bite)

- Calories: 110
- Protein: 9 g
- Carbs: 9 g (Fiber: 1 g)
- Fat: 5 g

Storage & Prep

- Refrigerate up to 5 days.
- Freeze up to 2 months.

# Chocolate Protein Pudding Cups

Servings: 4 | Prep Time: 10 min | Chill Time: 1 hr | Total Time: 1 hr 10 min
Icons: 🌱 Plant-Based option ❄ Freezer-Friendly

### Ingredients

- 2 cups unsweetened almond milk (or dairy milk)
- ½ cup chocolate protein powder
- 2 tbsp cocoa powder
- 2 tbsp cornstarch
- 1 tbsp maple syrup (optional)

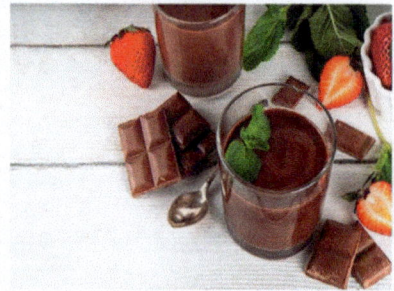

### Directions

1. Whisk almond milk, protein powder, cocoa, cornstarch, and maple syrup in saucepan.
2. Cook over medium heat until thickened.
3. Pour into cups and chill 1 hour.

Nutrition (per serving)

- Calories: 140
- Protein: 12 g
- Carbs: 15 g (Fiber: 3 g)
- Fat: 3 g

Storage & Prep

- Refrigerate up to 4 days.
- Freeze in single-serve containers up to 1 month.

# Almond Butter Protein Cookies

Servings: 12 cookies  |  Prep Time: 10 min  |  Cook Time: 12 min  |  Total Time: 22 min
Icons: 🌱 Plant-Based option  ⏱ Under 30 Min  ❄️ Freezer-Friendly

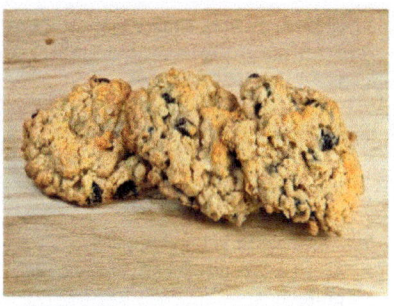

## Ingredients

- 1 cup rolled oats
- ½ cup vanilla protein powder
- ¼ cup almond butter
- ¼ cup honey or maple syrup
- ¼ cup raisins
- 1 egg (or flax egg)
- ½ tsp cinnamon

### Nutrition (per cookie)

- Calories: 120
- Protein: 8 g
- Carbs: 16 g (Fiber: 3 g)
- Fat: 5 g

## Directions

1. Preheat oven to 350°F (175°C).
2. Mix oats, protein powder, almond butter, syrup, egg, raisins, and cinnamon.
3. Scoop onto baking sheet; bake 10–12 minutes.

### Storage & Prep

- Refrigerate up to 5 days.
- Freeze up to 2 months.

# Greek Yogurt Chocolate Mousse

Servings: 2  |  Prep Time: 5 min  |  Chill Time: 30 min  |  Total Time: 35 min
Icons: ⏱ Under 30 Min

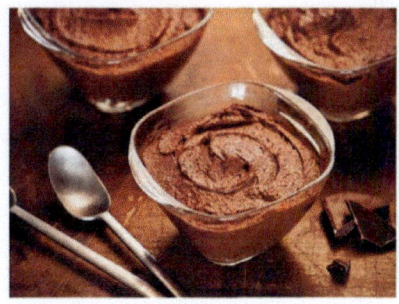

## Ingredients

- 1 cup plain Greek yogurt
- 2 tbsp cocoa powder
- 2 tbsp chocolate protein powder
- 1 tbsp maple syrup or honey
- ½ tsp vanilla extract

## Directions

1. Mix yogurt, cocoa, protein powder, syrup, and vanilla until creamy.
2. Chill 30 minutes before serving.

### Nutrition (per serving)

- Calories: 180
- Protein: 18 g
- Carbs: 14 g (Fiber: 3 g)
- Fat: 4 g

### Storage & Prep

- Refrigerate up to 3 days.
- Not freezer-friendly.

# Protein Mug Cake (90 Seconds)

Servings: 1 | Prep Time: 2 min | Cook
Time: 1.5 min | Total Time: 3.5 min
Icons: ⏱ Under 30 Min

### Ingredients

- 1 scoop chocolate or vanilla protein powder
- 2 tbsp oat flour (or almond flour)
- 1 tbsp cocoa powder (if using vanilla protein)
- ¼ tsp baking powder
- 1 egg white (or flax egg)
- 3 tbsp almond milk

### Directions

1. Mix all ingredients in a mug until smooth.
2. Microwave 90 seconds until cooked through.

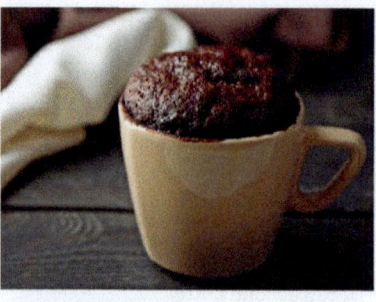

Nutrition (per serving)

- Calories: 220
- Protein: 22 g
- Carbs: 18 g (Fiber: 4 g)
- Fat: 6 g

Storage & Prep

- Best eaten fresh.
- Batter can be prepped dry in jars for quick use.

# Peanut Butter Protein Fudge

Servings: 12 small squares | Prep Time: 10
min | Chill Time: 1 hr | Total Time: 1 hr
10 min
Icons: 🌱 Plant-Based option ❄ Freezer-Friendly

### Ingredients

- 1 cup natural peanut butter
- ½ cup vanilla protein powder
- ¼ cup coconut oil, melted
- 2 tbsp maple syrup
- 1 tsp vanilla extract

### Directions

1. Mix all ingredients until smooth.
2. Spread into parchment-lined pan.
3. Chill 1 hour, then cut into squares.

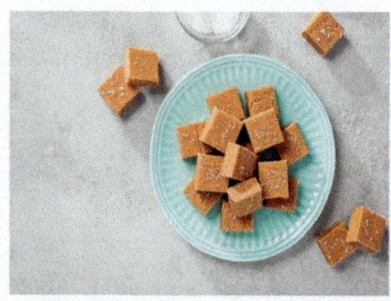

Nutrition (per square)

- Calories: 120
- Protein: 7 g
- Carbs: 6 g (Fiber: 1 g)
- Fat: 9 g

Storage & Prep

- Refrigerate up to 1 week.
- Freeze up to 2 months.

# High-Protein Banana Bread

Servings: 10 slices | Prep Time: 15 min | Cook Time: 40 min | Total Time: 55 min
Icons: 🌱 Plant-Based option ❄️ Freezer-Friendly

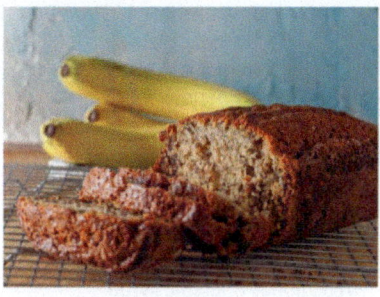

### Ingredients

- 2 ripe bananas, mashed
- 1 cup oat flour
- ½ cup vanilla protein powder
- 2 eggs (or flax eggs for vegan)
- 2 tbsp honey or maple syrup
- 1 tsp baking powder
- 1 tsp cinnamon

### Directions

1. Preheat oven to 350°F (175°C).
2. Mix bananas, eggs, and syrup. Stir in flour, protein powder, baking powder, and cinnamon.
3. Pour into loaf pan and bake 35–40 minutes.

**Nutrition (per slice)**

- Calories: 140
- Protein: 10 g
- Carbs: 20 g (Fiber: 3 g)
- Fat: 4 g

**Storage & Prep**

- Refrigerate up to 5 days.
- Freeze slices up to 2 months.

# Mocha Protein Smoothie Pops

Servings: 6 popsicles | Prep Time: 5 min | Freeze Time: 4 hrs | Total Time: 4 hrs+
Icons: 🌱 Plant-Based option ❄️ Freezer-Friendly

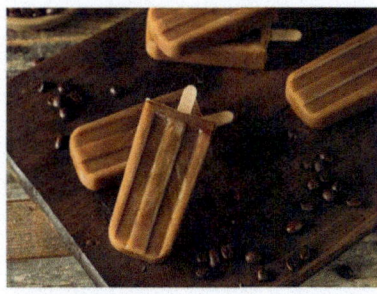

### Ingredients

- 2 cups unsweetened almond milk
- 1 scoop chocolate protein powder
- 1 tsp instant coffee granules
- 1 tbsp cocoa powder
- 1 tbsp maple syrup (optional)

### Directions

1. Blend all ingredients until smooth.
2. Pour into popsicle molds and freeze at least 4 hours.

**Nutrition (per pop)**

- Calories: 80
- Protein: 7 g
- Carbs: 9 g (Fiber: 2 g)
- Fat: 2 g

**Storage & Prep**

- Keep frozen up to 2 months.
- Run molds under warm water to release pops.

# Protein Oatmeal Raisin Cookies

Servings: 12 cookies  |  Prep Time: 10 min  |  Cook Time: 12 min  |  Total Time: 22 min
Icons: 🌱 Plant-Based option  ⏱ Under 30 Min  ❄️ Freezer-Friendly

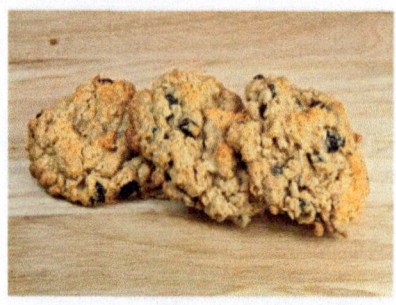

### Ingredients

- 1 cup rolled oats
- ½ cup vanilla protein powder
- ¼ cup almond butter
- ¼ cup honey or maple syrup
- ¼ cup raisins
- 1 egg (or flax egg)
- ½ tsp cinnamon

**Nutrition (per cookie)**

- Calories: 120
- Protein: 8 g
- Carbs: 16 g (Fiber: 3 g)
- Fat: 5 g

### Directions

1. Preheat oven to 350°F (175°C).
2. Mix oats, protein powder, almond butter, syrup, egg, raisins, and cinnamon.
3. Scoop onto baking sheet; bake 10–12 minutes.

**Storage & Prep**

- Refrigerate up to 5 days.
- Freeze up to 2 months.

# Vanilla Protein Ice Cream

Servings: 4  |  Prep Time: 10 min  |  Freeze Time: 2 hrs  |  Total Time: 2 hrs 10 min
Icons: 🌱 Plant-Based option  ❄️ Freezer-Friendly

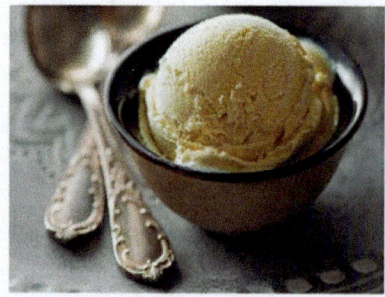

### Ingredients

- 2 cups unsweetened almond milk
- 1 scoop vanilla protein powder
- 1 frozen banana
- 1 tsp vanilla extract
- 1 tbsp maple syrup (optional)

**Nutrition (per serving)**

- Calories: 130
- Protein: 11 g
- Carbs: 18 g (Fiber: 4 g)
- Fat: 3 g

### Directions

1. Blend all ingredients until creamy.
2. Pour into freezer-safe container.
3. Freeze 2 hours, stirring every 30 minutes for soft-serve texture.

**Storage & Prep**

- Store frozen up to 2 weeks.
- Thaw 5 minutes before scooping.

# Strawberry Protein Cheesecake Parfaits

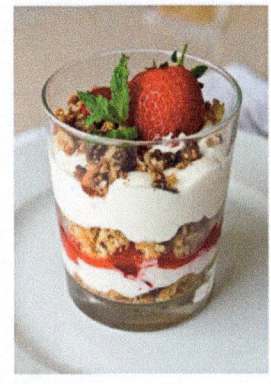

Servings: 4  |  Prep Time: 10 min  |  Chill Time: 30 min  |  Total Time: 40 min
Icons: 🌱 Plant-Based option  🕐 Under 30 Min

## Ingredients

- 1 cup low-fat cream cheese (or dairy-free alternative)
- ½ cup Greek yogurt
- ½ cup vanilla protein powder
- 1 cup crushed graham crackers (or almond flour for GF)
- 1 cup sliced strawberries
- 1 tbsp honey or maple syrup

## Directions

1. Whisk cream cheese, yogurt, protein powder, and honey until smooth.
2. Layer graham crumbs, cheesecake filling, and strawberries in cups.
3. Chill 30 minutes before serving.

**Nutrition (per serving)**

- Calories: 210
- Protein: 16 g
- Carbs: 23 g (Fiber: 3 g)
- Fat: 7 g

**Storage & Prep**

- Refrigerate up to 3 days.
- Not freezer-friendly.

# Double Chocolate Protein Brownies

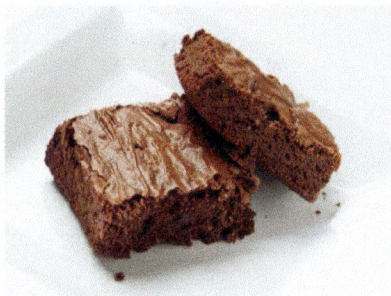

Servings: 9 squares  |  Prep Time: 10 min  |  Cook Time: 20 min  |  Total Time: 30 min
Icons: 🌱 Plant-Based option  ❄️ Freezer-Friendly

## Ingredients

- 1 cup oat flour
- ½ cup chocolate protein powder
- ¼ cup cocoa powder
- ½ cup unsweetened applesauce
- ¼ cup almond butter
- ¼ cup maple syrup
- 1 tsp baking powder
- ¼ cup dark chocolate chips

## Directions

1. Preheat oven to 350°F (175°C). Line baking pan.
2. Mix all ingredients into smooth batter.
3. Spread in pan and bake 18–20 minutes.
4. Cool before slicing into squares.

**Nutrition (per square)**

- Calories: 150
- Protein: 10 g
- Carbs: 20 g (Fiber: 4 g)
- Fat: 6 g

**Storage & Prep**

- Store in airtight container up to 4 days.
- Freeze brownies up to 2 months.

# Part
# III
# Specialized Tracks

# Chapter 10

# Budget & Batch Cooking

◆

Eating high-protein doesn't have to be expensive—or exhausting. In this chapter, you'll learn how to stretch your grocery budget while still hitting your protein goals, using smart shopping strategies and batch-cooking techniques that save both time and money.

You'll find 12 recipes designed for bulk prep, freezer storage, and family-style portions. These include hearty stews, sheet-pan meals, and versatile proteins that can be repurposed across multiple dishes during the week. Alongside the recipes, you'll also get practical tools and tips for meal planning, shopping, and storage so you can make your protein dollars go further.

This chapter is about more than recipes—it's about creating a system you can sustain. With a little planning, you'll discover that high-protein eating can be simple, affordable, and stress-free.

# Budget-Friendly Tools & Strategies

Cooking high-protein meals on a budget is all about working smarter, not harder. By investing in a few reliable tools and using simple strategies, you can cut costs, reduce waste, and make meal prep much easier.

## Essential Tools

- **Slow Cooker or Instant Pot:** Perfect for large-batch stews, beans, and shredded meats. They turn inexpensive cuts of meat or dry legumes into tender, protein-rich meals.

- **Sheet Pans & Casserole Dishes:** Ideal for roasting in bulk— whether it's chicken, tofu, or trays of vegetables. Minimal cleanup, maximum yield.

- **Sharp Knives & Cutting Boards:** Prepping in bulk is faster and safer with a good set of knives and durable boards.

- **Freezer-Safe Containers & Bags:** Investing in reusable, stackable containers makes portioning and storing large batches easy.

## Smart Strategies

- **Buy in Bulk:** Proteins like chicken breast, ground turkey, lentils, beans, and tofu are often cheaper in family packs or warehouse stores. Divide and freeze for later use.

- **Plan Once, Cook Twice:** Choose versatile base proteins—like roasted chicken, chili, or lentils—that can be repurposed into wraps, bowls, or salads.

- **Season Creatively, Not Expensively:** Budget-friendly pantry staples (cumin, paprika, garlic powder, soy sauce) can transform the same protein into different flavor profiles throughout the week.

- **Freeze Wisely:** Label meals with the date and type so nothing gets lost. Freeze in single portions for quick grab-and-go meals.

- Batch **Prep Snacks Too:** Boiled eggs, roasted chickpeas, and protein muffins are low-cost snacks that can be made in bulk and stored for days.

By pairing the right tools with these strategies, you'll discover that eating high-protein on a budget isn't about restriction—it's about efficiency and creativity.

Here's a $7/day high-protein weekly menu designed to be budget-friendly while still hitting strong protein goals. Costs are approximate based on bulk/discount grocery averages in the U.S.

# Daily Structure (~$7/day)

- **Breakfast:** $1.50
- **Snack:** $0.75–$1.00
- **Lunch:** $2.00
- **Snack:** $0.75–$1.00
- **Dinner:** $2.00

# 7-Day Sample Menu

## Day 1

- **Breakfast:** Overnight oats with whey protein + peanut butter ($1.50)
- **Snack:** 2 boiled eggs + carrot sticks ($0.80)
- **Lunch:** Lentil & tuna salad with olive oil + lemon ($2.00)
- **Snack:** Cottage cheese with pineapple chunks ($0.90)
- **Dinner:** Sheet-pan chicken thighs with broccoli + sweet potato ($2.00)

## Day 2

- **Breakfast:** Greek yogurt with frozen berries + scoop protein powder ($1.50)

- **Snack:** Roasted chickpeas (homemade) ($0.75)

- **Lunch:** Turkey & black bean burrito bowl ($2.00)

- **Snack:** Peanut butter on whole wheat toast ($0.80)

- **Dinner:** Egg + veggie fried "rice" with frozen peas and tofu ($2.00)

**Day 3**

- **Breakfast:** Protein pancakes (oats, egg, protein powder) ($1.50)

- **Snack:** Edamame with sea salt ($0.90)

- **Lunch:** Chicken chili with beans + corn ($2.00)

- **Snack:** Protein smoothie with banana + milk ($1.00)

- **Dinner:** Baked salmon with rice + green beans ($2.00, bulk frozen salmon)

**Day 4**

- **Breakfast:** Cottage cheese + sliced apple + cinnamon ($1.40)

- **Snack:** Hard-boiled eggs + cucumber sticks ($0.80)

- **Lunch:** Lentil & quinoa Buddha bowl with roasted veggies ($2.00)

- **Snack:** High-protein hummus with celery ($0.90)

- **Dinner:** Ground turkey stir-fry with cabbage + carrots ($2.00)

**Day 5**

- **Breakfast:** Scrambled eggs with spinach + whole wheat toast ($1.50)

- **Snack:** Greek yogurt parfait with granola ($1.00)

- **Lunch:** Tuna wrap with lettuce + chickpeas ($2.00)

- **Snack:** Almonds (1 oz) + protein shake ($1.00)

- **Dinner:** Slow cooker pulled BBQ chicken with rice ($2.00)

## Day 6

- **Breakfast:** Protein mug cake (90 sec) with banana slices ($1.50)

- **Snack:** Roasted edamame ($0.90)

- **Lunch:** Turkey & lentil soup with carrots + celery ($2.00)

- **Snack:** Apple slices + peanut butter ($0.80)

- **Dinner:** One-pan baked cod with roasted sweet potato + broccoli ($2.00)

## Day 7

- **Breakfast:** High-protein smoothie (milk, oats, protein powder, berries) ($1.50)

- **Snack:** Cottage cheese with sliced cucumber ($0.80)

- **Lunch:** Black bean & quinoa salad with avocado ($2.00)

- **Snack:** Protein balls (oats, peanut butter, protein powder) ($0.90)

- **Dinner:** Chicken + vegetable curry with rice ($2.00)

- **Macros:** Each day provides ~100–120g protein, balanced carbs, and healthy fats.
- **Budget:** $7 per day ($49/week).
- **Batch-Friendly:** Lentils, beans, rice, chicken, and eggs are cooked in bulk and reused across multiple days to save time and money.

# Recipe Icons Guide

🔍 **One-Pan**
Cook the whole meal in a single pan — less cleanup, more convenience.

❄️ **Freezer-Friendly**
Can be stored in the freezer for later; reheats well.

$ **Budget-Friendly**
Costs under $4 per serving with common ingredients.

⏱️ **Under 30 Minutes**
From prep to plate in half an hour or less.

⭐ **30+ g Protein**
Each serving delivers at least 30 grams of protein.

🌱 **Plant-Based**
Fully vegetarian or vegan protein sources.

# Big-Batch Turkey & Veggie Meatballs

Servings: 24 meatballs (6 servings)  |  Prep Time: 20 min  |  Cook Time: 25 min  |  Total Time: 45 min
Icons: $ Budget-Friendly  ❄ Freezer-Friendly  🔍 One-Pan

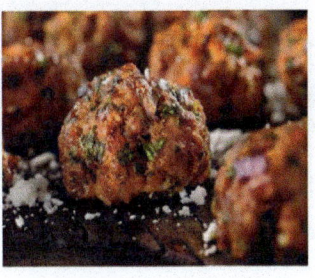

## Ingredients

- 2 lbs ground turkey
- 1 cup breadcrumbs (or oats)
- 1 cup grated zucchini or carrot
- 2 eggs
- 2 tsp garlic powder
- 1 tsp salt
- 1 tsp black pepper

**Nutrition (per serving = 4 meatballs)**

- Calories: 240
- Protein: 27 g
- Carbs: 12 g (Fiber: 2 g)
- Fat: 9 g

## Directions

1. Preheat oven to 375°F (190°C). Line baking sheet.
2. Mix turkey, breadcrumbs, veggies, eggs, and seasonings.
3. Roll into 24 meatballs; place on baking sheet.
4. Bake 20–25 minutes until cooked through.

**Storage & Prep**

- Refrigerate up to 4 days.
- Freeze up to 3 months; reheat from frozen in sauce or oven.

# Slow Cooker Bean & Beef Chili

Servings: 8  |  Prep Time: 15 min  |  Cook Time: 6–8 hrs  |  Total Time: 8 hrs+
Icons: $ Budget-Friendly  ❄ Freezer-Friendly  🔍 One-Pot

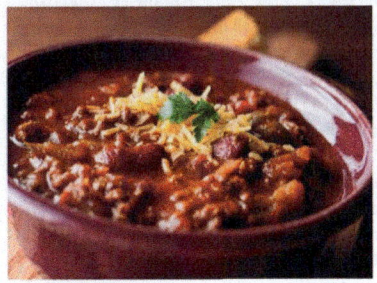

## Ingredients

- 1 lb lean ground beef
- 2 cans (15 oz each) kidney beans, drained
- 2 cans (15 oz each) black beans, drained
- 1 can (28 oz) crushed tomatoes
- 1 onion, diced
- 1 bell pepper, diced
- 2 tbsp chili powder
- 1 tsp cumin
- Salt & pepper, to taste

**Nutrition (per serving)**

- Calories: 310
- Protein: 28 g
- Carbs: 32 g (Fiber: 10 g)
- Fat: 9 g

## Directions

1. Brown beef in skillet. Transfer to slow cooker.
2. Add beans, tomatoes, onion, pepper, and spices.
3. Cook on low 6–8 hrs (or high 4 hrs).

**Storage & Prep**

- Refrigerate up to 5 days.
- Freeze in portions up to 3 months.

# Bulk Overnight Oats (5-Day Prep)

Servings: 5 jars  |  Prep Time: 10 min  |
Total Time: 10 min + chill overnight
Icons: $ Budget-Friendly  ❄ Freezer-
Friendly option  ⏱ Under 30 Min

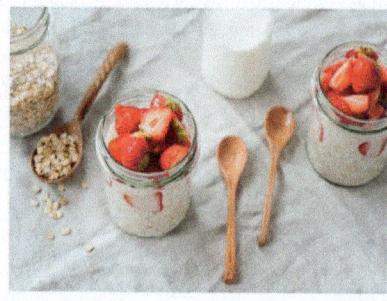

### Ingredients (per jar)

- ½ cup rolled oats
- ½ cup milk (dairy or plant-based)
- ½ cup Greek yogurt
- 1 scoop vanilla protein powder
- ½ cup frozen berries

### Directions

1. Mix oats, milk, yogurt, and protein powder in jars.
2. Top with berries.
3. Chill overnight.

### Nutrition (per jar)

- Calories: 320
- Protein: 28 g
- Carbs: 40 g (Fiber: 7 g)
- Fat: 5 g

### Storage & Prep

- Refrigerate up to 5 days.
- Can freeze without fruit topping up to 1 month.

# Sheet-Pan Chicken & Veggies (4 Meals in 1 Pan)

Servings: 4  |  Prep Time: 10 min  |  Cook Time: 25 min  |  Total Time: 35 min
Icons: $ Budget-Friendly  🔍 One-Pan  ⏱ Under 30 Min

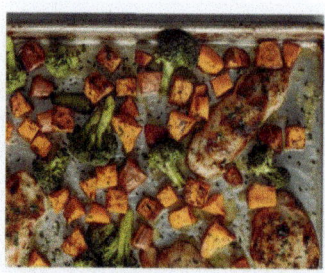

### Ingredients

- 4 chicken breasts (about 2 lbs)
- 2 cups broccoli florets
- 2 cups diced sweet potatoes
- 2 tbsp olive oil
- 1 tsp paprika
- 1 tsp garlic powder
- Salt & pepper, to taste

### Directions

1. Preheat oven to 400°F (200°C).
2. Spread chicken, broccoli, and sweet potatoes on sheet pan.
3. Drizzle with oil and seasonings.
4. Bake 25 minutes until chicken is cooked and veggies are tender.

### Nutrition (per serving)

- Calories: 370
- Protein: 38 g
- Carbs: 28 g (Fiber: 6 g)
- Fat: 11 g

### Storage & Prep

- Refrigerate up to 4 days.
- Portion into meal-prep containers for grab-and-go lunches/dinners.

# Big-Batch Lentil & Veggie Soup

Servings: 8  |  Prep Time: 15 min  |  Cook Time: 40 min  |  Total Time: 55 min
Icons: 🌱 Plant-Based  💲 Budget-Friendly  🍲 One-Pot  ❄️ Freezer-Friendly

## Ingredients

- 2 cups dry lentils, rinsed
- 1 onion, diced
- 2 carrots, diced
- 2 celery stalks, diced
- 1 can (28 oz) crushed tomatoes
- 6 cups vegetable broth
- 2 tsp Italian seasoning
- Salt & pepper, to taste

## Directions

1. Sauté onion, carrots, and celery 5 minutes.
2. Add lentils, tomatoes, broth, and seasoning.
3. Simmer 35–40 minutes until lentils are tender.

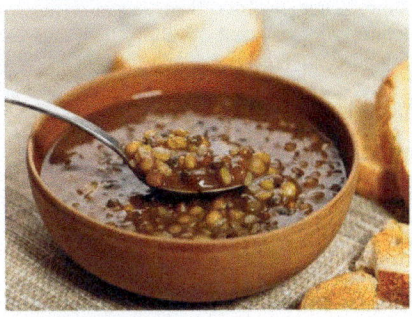

Nutrition (per serving)

- Calories: 250
- Protein: 18 g
- Carbs: 42 g (Fiber: 12 g)
- Fat: 2 g

Storage & Prep

- Refrigerate up to 5 days.
- Freeze in portions up to 3 months.

# Bulk Egg & Veggie Muffins

Servings: 12 muffins (6 servings)  |  Prep Time: 10 min  |  Cook Time: 20 min  |  Total Time: 30 min
Icons: 💲 Budget-Friendly  ⏱️ Under 30 Min  ❄️ Freezer-Friendly

## Ingredients

- 12 eggs
- 1 cup diced bell peppers
- 1 cup spinach, chopped
- ½ cup shredded cheddar cheese
- 1 tsp salt
- ½ tsp black pepper

## Directions

1. Preheat oven to 375°F (190°C). Grease muffin tin.
2. Whisk eggs with salt and pepper. Stir in veggies and cheese.
3. Pour into muffin cups; bake 18–20 minutes until set.

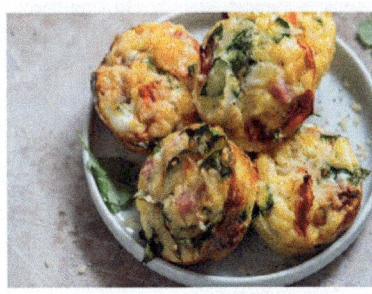

Nutrition (per serving = 2 muffins)

- Calories: 190
- Protein: 16 g
- Carbs: 3 g (Fiber: 1 g)
- Fat: 12 g

Storage & Prep

- Refrigerate up to 5 days.
- Freeze up to 2 months.

# Big-Batch Black Bean & Quinoa Bowls

Servings: 6 | Prep Time: 15 min | Cook Time: 20 min | Total Time: 35 min
Icons: 🌱 Plant-Based  $ Budget-Friendly  ❄ Freezer-Friendly

### Ingredients

- 2 cups dry quinoa
- 3 cans (15 oz each) black beans, rinsed
- 1 onion, diced
- 2 bell peppers, diced
- 2 tsp cumin
- 1 tsp chili powder
- 2 tbsp olive oil

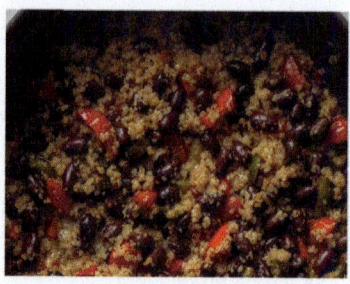

### Directions

1. Cook quinoa according to package.
2. In skillet, sauté onion and peppers in olive oil.
3. Stir in black beans, quinoa, and spices.

### Nutrition (per serving)

- Calories: 360
- Protein: 19 g
- Carbs: 54 g (Fiber: 12 g)
- Fat: 9 g

### Storage & Prep

- Refrigerate up to 5 days.
- Freeze in portions up to 2 months.

# Family-Size Chicken & Rice Casserole

Servings: 8 | Prep Time: 15 min | Cook Time: 45 min | Total Time: 1 hr
Icons: $ Budget-Friendly  🔍 One-Pan  ❄ Freezer-Friendly

### Ingredients

- 2 lbs boneless, skinless chicken thighs
- 2 cups uncooked rice
- 4 cups chicken broth
- 1 onion, diced
- 1 cup frozen peas
- 1 cup shredded cheddar
- 1 tsp garlic powder
- 1 tsp paprika

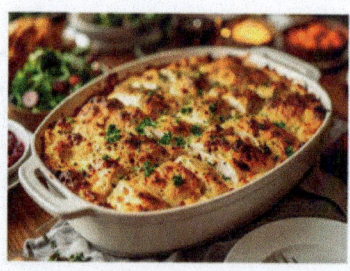

### Directions

1. Preheat oven to 375°F (190°C).
2. Layer rice, broth, onion, peas, and spices in casserole dish.
3. Place chicken thighs on top; cover with foil.
4. Bake 40–45 minutes until rice and chicken are fully cooked.
5. Sprinkle cheese before serving.

### Nutrition (per serving)

- Calories: 400
- Protein: 31 g
- Carbs: 42 g (Fiber: 3 g)
- Fat: 12 g

### Storage & Prep

- Refrigerate up to 4 days.
- Freeze in portions up to 3 months.

# Big-Batch Turkey & Lentil Sloppy Joes

Servings: 8  |  Prep Time: 15 min  |  Cook Time: 30 min  |  Total Time: 45 min
Icons: $ Budget-Friendly  🍲 One-Pot  ❄️ Freezer-Friendly

## Ingredients

- 1 lb ground turkey
- 1 cup dry lentils, rinsed
- 1 can (15 oz) tomato sauce
- 1 onion, diced
- 1 bell pepper, diced
- 2 tbsp ketchup
- 1 tbsp Worcestershire sauce
- 2 tsp chili powder

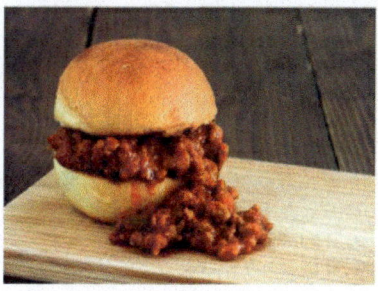

## Directions

1. Cook lentils in 3 cups water until tender, about 20 minutes.
2. Brown turkey in skillet; add onion, pepper, and seasonings.
3. Stir in lentils and tomato sauce. Simmer 10 minutes.

### Nutrition (per serving)

- Calories: 290
- Protein: 26 g
- Carbs: 34 g (Fiber: 8 g)
- Fat: 7 g

### Storage & Prep

- Refrigerate up to 4 days.
- Freeze filling up to 2 months.

# Bulk-Buy Rotisserie Chicken Meal Prep

Servings: 5  |  Prep Time: 20 min  |  Total Time: 20 min
Icons: $ Budget-Friendly  🕐 Under 30 Min

## Ingredients

- 1 store-bought rotisserie chicken
- 3 cups cooked brown rice
- 3 cups steamed broccoli
- 1 cup shredded carrots
- ½ cup low-sodium soy sauce

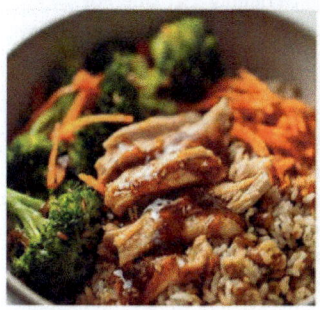

## Directions

1. Shred chicken and divide into 5 containers.
2. Add rice, broccoli, and carrots.
3. Drizzle with soy sauce before serving.

### Nutrition (per serving)

- Calories: 420
- Protein: 35 g
- Carbs: 42 g (Fiber: 6 g)
- Fat: 11 g

### Storage & Prep

- Refrigerate up to 4 days.
- Best eaten fresh (rotisserie chicken doesn't freeze well).

# Big-Batch Egg Fried Rice

Servings: 6 | Prep Time: 15 min | Cook Time: 15 min | Total Time: 30 min
Icons: $ Budget-Friendly 🔍 One-Pan ⏱ Under 30 Min

### Ingredients

- 4 cups cooked rice (day-old works best)
- 6 eggs, beaten
- 2 cups frozen peas & carrots
- 3 tbsp soy sauce
- 1 tbsp sesame oil
- 2 green onions, sliced

### Directions

1. Heat sesame oil in large skillet.
2. Add peas and carrots; cook 5 minutes.
3. Push veggies aside; scramble eggs.
4. Stir in rice, soy sauce, and green onions.

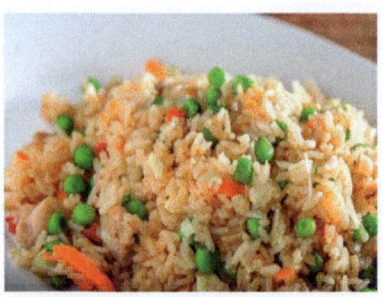

### Nutrition (per serving)

- Calories: 310
- Protein: 15 g
- Carbs: 42 g (Fiber: 4 g)
- Fat: 10 g

### Storage & Prep

- Refrigerate up to 5 days.
- Freeze portions up to 2 months.

# Freezer-Friendly Beef & Veggie Stew

Servings: 8 | Prep Time: 20 min | Cook Time: 1 hr | Total Time: 1 hr 20 min
Icons: $ Budget-Friendly 🔍 One-Pot ❄ Freezer-Friendly

### Ingredients

- 2 lbs beef stew meat
- 4 carrots, sliced
- 3 potatoes, cubed
- 1 onion, diced
- 4 cups beef broth
- 2 tbsp tomato paste
- 2 tsp thyme
- 1 bay leaf
- Salt & pepper, to taste

### Directions

1. Brown beef in pot.
2. Add carrots, potatoes, onion, broth, tomato paste, and seasonings.
3. Bring to boil; reduce heat and simmer 1 hour until tender.

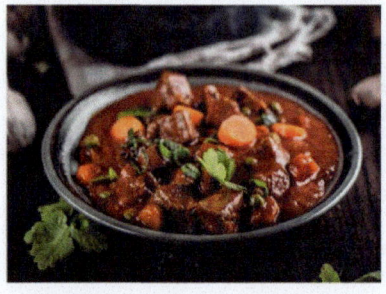

### Nutrition (per serving)

- Calories: 390
- Protein: 34 g
- Carbs: 28 g (Fiber: 4 g)
- Fat: 15 g

### Storage & Prep

- Refrigerate up to 4 days.
- Freeze up to 3 months.

# Chapter 11

# GLP-1 Friendly High-Protein Meals

✦

If you're using a GLP-1 medication like semaglutide (Ozempic®), tirzepatide (Mounjaro®), or similar, you know that appetite often decreases—but your nutrition needs do not. In fact, eating enough protein becomes even more important to maintain lean muscle, support steady energy, and avoid nutrient gaps.

This chapter is designed specifically with GLP-1 users in mind. You'll find meals that are **high in protein, gentle on digestion, portion-friendly, and simple to prepare.** Each recipe focuses on lean protein sources, fiber-rich vegetables, and balanced healthy fats to maximize satiety without overwhelming your appetite.

With 11 recipes, you'll learn how to:

- Pack in protein even with smaller meals.

- Choose foods that support muscle and metabolism during weight loss.

- Build meals that are satisfying without being heavy.

- Prep in advance so you're never stuck with choices that don't fit your goals.

Whether you're looking for smooth, soft-textured meals that are easy to tolerate, or flavorful, nutrient-dense dishes in smaller portions, this chapter gives you practical, GLP-1–friendly options that align with your high-protein lifestyle.

# Recipe Icons Guide

🔍 **One-Pan**
Cook the whole meal in a single pan —
less cleanup, more convenience.

⏱ **Under 30 Minutes**
From prep to plate in half an hour or
less.

❄️ **Freezer-Friendly**
Can be stored in the freezer for later;
reheats well.

⭐ **30+ g Protein**
Each serving delivers at least 30 grams
of protein.

$ **Budget-Friendly**
Costs under $4 per serving with
common ingredients.

🌱 **Plant-Based**
Fully vegetarian or vegan protein
sources.

# Soft Scrambled Eggs with Cottage Cheese

Servings: 1  |  Prep Time: 5 min  |  Cook Time: 5 min  |  Total Time: 10 min
Icons: ⏱ Under 30 Min    $ Budget-Friendly

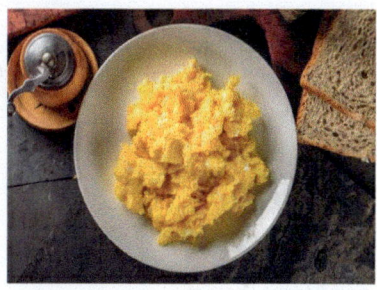

## Ingredients

- 2 large eggs
- ¼ cup low-fat cottage cheese
- 1 tsp olive oil or butter
- Salt & pepper, to taste

## Directions

1. Whisk eggs and cottage cheese together until smooth.
2. Heat oil in nonstick skillet on low.
3. Pour mixture in and gently scramble until soft and creamy.

**Nutrition (per serving)**

- Calories: 220
- Protein: 22 g
- Carbs: 3 g
- Fat: 13 g

**Storage & Prep**

- Best eaten fresh.
- Not freezer-friendly.

# Mini Salmon Patties

Servings: 4 (8 patties)  |  Prep Time: 10 min  |  Cook Time: 10 min  |  Total Time: 20 min
Icons: ⏱ Under 30 Min    ❄ Freezer-Friendly

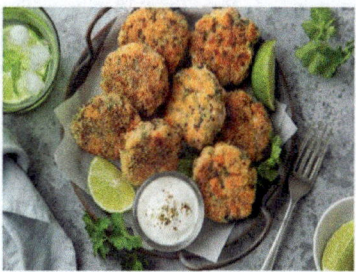

## Ingredients

- 2 cans (5 oz each) salmon, drained
- 1 egg
- ¼ cup breadcrumbs (or almond flour for GF)
- 1 tbsp Greek yogurt
- 1 tsp lemon juice

## Directions

1. Mix all ingredients in a bowl.
2. Form into 8 small patties.
3. Cook in lightly oiled skillet, 3–4 min per side.

**Nutrition (per serving = 2 patties)**

- Calories: 190
- Protein: 22 g
- Carbs: 4 g
- Fat: 9 g

**Storage & Prep**

- Refrigerate up to 3 days.
- Freeze cooked patties up to 2 months.

# Greek Yogurt Protein Smoothie

Servings: 1 | Prep Time: 5 min | Total Time: 5 min
Icons: 🌱 Plant-Based option ⏱ Under 30 Min

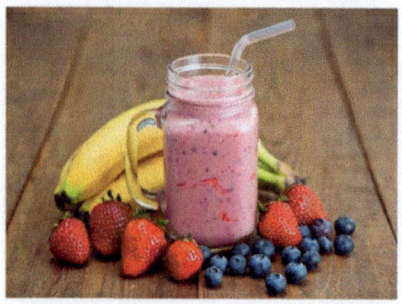

## Ingredients

- ½ cup Greek yogurt
- ½ cup milk (dairy or plant-based)
- 1 scoop protein powder
- ½ banana (frozen)
- ½ cup frozen berries

## Directions

1. Blend all ingredients until smooth.
2. Add water to thin if needed.

### Nutrition (per serving)

- Calories: 280
- Protein: 30 g
- Carbs: 28 g (Fiber: 5 g)
- Fat: 5 g

### Storage & Prep

- Best consumed fresh.
- Can pre-bag fruit + powder for freezer packs.

# Soft Tofu & Veggie Stir-Fry

Servings: 2 | Prep Time: 10 min | Cook Time: 10 min | Total Time: 20 min
Icons: 🌱 Plant-Based 🍳 One-Pan ⏱ Under 30 Min

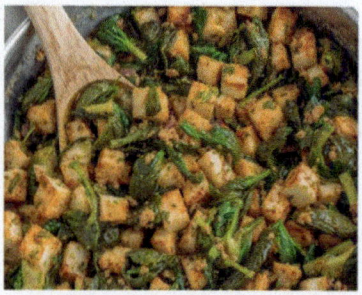

## Ingredients

- 8 oz soft tofu, cubed
- 1 cup zucchini, diced
- 1 cup spinach
- 1 tbsp soy sauce
- 1 tsp sesame oil

## Directions

1. Heat sesame oil in skillet.
2. Add zucchini and cook 3 minutes.
3. Gently stir in tofu, soy sauce, and spinach until warmed through.

### Nutrition (per serving)

- Calories: 190
- Protein: 17 g
- Carbs: 8 g
- Fat: 9 g

### Storage & Prep

- Refrigerate up to 2 days.
- Not freezer-friendly.

# Chicken & Lentil Soup (Easy Digest)

Servings: 4 | Prep Time: 10 min | Cook
Time: 30 min | Total Time: 40 min
Icons: $ Budget-Friendly 🔍 One-Pot ❄️
Freezer-Friendly

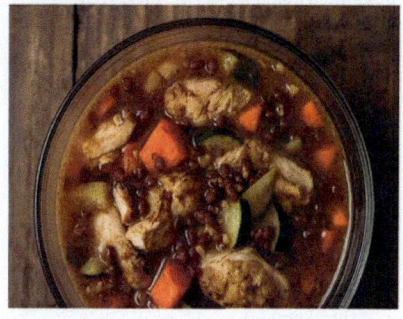

## Ingredients

- 1 lb chicken breast, cubed
- 1 cup red lentils, rinsed
- 1 carrot, diced
- 1 zucchini, diced
- 6 cups chicken broth
- 1 tsp turmeric
- ½ tsp salt

**Nutrition (per serving)**

- Calories: 250
- Protein: 28 g
- Carbs: 18 g (Fiber: 6 g)
- Fat: 6 g

## Directions

1. In large pot, simmer chicken and broth 10 minutes.
2. Add lentils, carrot, zucchini, and turmeric.
3. Cook 20 minutes until lentils are soft.

**Storage & Prep**

- Refrigerate up to 4 days.
- Freeze in portions up to 2 months.

# Egg White & Spinach Omelet

Servings: 1 | Prep Time: 5 min | Cook
Time: 5 min | Total Time: 10 min
Icons: ⏱️ Under 30 Min $ Budget-Friendly

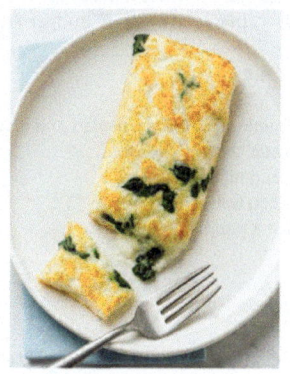

## Ingredients

- 4 egg whites
- ½ cup chopped spinach
- 2 tbsp shredded mozzarella
- Salt & pepper, to taste

**Nutrition (per serving)**

- Calories: 130
- Protein: 20 g
- Carbs: 2 g
- Fat: 4 g

## Directions

1. Whisk egg whites with salt and pepper.
2. Heat nonstick skillet; add spinach and cook 1–2 minutes.
3. Pour in egg whites; cook until set. Sprinkle cheese before folding.

**Storage & Prep**

- Best eaten fresh.
- Not freezer-friendly.

# Turkey & Zucchini Mini Meatloaves

Servings: 6 mini loaves | Prep Time: 15 min | Cook Time: 25 min | Total Time: 40 min
Icons: $ Budget-Friendly ❄ Freezer-Friendly

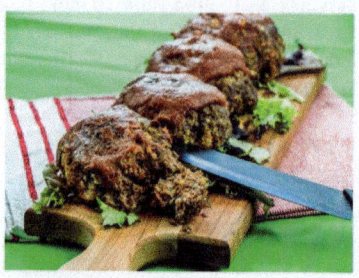

## Ingredients

- 1 lb ground turkey
- 1 cup grated zucchini
- ½ cup breadcrumbs (or oats)
- 1 egg
- 2 tbsp ketchup
- 1 tsp garlic powder

## Directions

1. Preheat oven to 375°F (190°C).
2. Mix turkey, zucchini, breadcrumbs, egg, ketchup, and seasoning.
3. Divide into muffin tin cups. Bake 25 minutes.

### Nutrition (per loaf)

- Calories: 140
- Protein: 16 g
- Carbs: 7 g
- Fat: 5 g

### Storage & Prep

- Refrigerate up to 4 days.
- Freeze up to 2 months.

# Creamy Protein Mashed Potatoes

Servings: 4 | Prep Time: 10 min | Cook Time: 15 min | Total Time: 25 min
Icons: ⏱ Under 30 Min $ Budget-Friendly

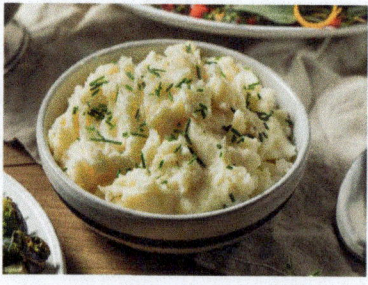

## Ingredients

- 4 medium potatoes, peeled and diced
- ½ cup cottage cheese
- ¼ cup milk
- 1 tbsp butter
- Salt & pepper, to taste

## Directions

1. Boil potatoes until fork-tender. Drain.
2. Mash with cottage cheese, milk, butter, salt, and pepper.
3. Blend with immersion blender for smoother texture, if desired.

### Nutrition (per serving)

- Calories: 210
- Protein: 14 g
- Carbs: 28 g (Fiber: 4 g)
- Fat: 6 g

### Storage & Prep

- Refrigerate up to 4 days.
- Freeze in single portions up to 1 month.

# Soft-Baked Cod with Lemon

Servings: 2  |  Prep Time: 5 min  |  Cook Time: 15 min  |  Total Time: 20 min
Icons: ⏱ Under 30 Min   $ Budget-Friendly   ❄ Freezer-Friendly

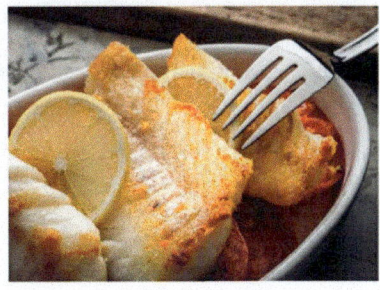

## Ingredients

- 2 cod fillets (about 6 oz each)
- 1 tbsp olive oil
- Juice of 1 lemon
- ½ tsp garlic powder
- ½ tsp paprika
- Salt & pepper, to taste

## Directions

1. Preheat oven to 375°F (190°C).
2. Place cod on baking sheet; drizzle with oil and lemon juice.
3. Sprinkle with seasonings; bake 12–15 minutes until flaky.

**Nutrition (per serving)**

- Calories: 210
- Protein: 28 g
- Carbs: 1 g
- Fat: 10 g

**Storage & Prep**

- Refrigerate up to 3 days.
- Freeze fillets up to 2 months.

# Protein-Packed Greek Yogurt Egg Salad

Servings: 3  |  Prep Time: 10 min  |  Total Time: 10 min
Icons: ⏱ Under 30 Min   $ Budget-Friendly

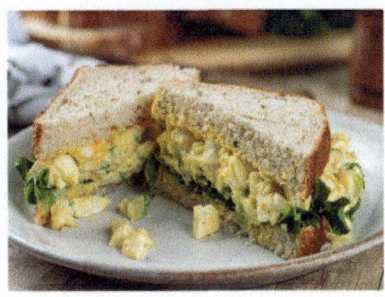

## Ingredients

- 6 hard-boiled eggs, chopped
- ½ cup Greek yogurt
- 1 tbsp Dijon mustard
- 1 tbsp chopped dill pickles
- Salt & pepper, to taste

## Directions

1. Mix chopped eggs, yogurt, mustard, pickles, salt, and pepper.
2. Serve on whole wheat toast or lettuce cups.

**Nutrition (per serving)**

- Calories: 210
- Protein: 19 g
- Carbs: 3 g
- Fat: 13 g

**Storage & Prep**

- Refrigerate up to 3 days.
- Not freezer-friendly.

# Cottage Cheese & Berry Protein Whip

Servings: 2 | Prep Time: 5 min | Total Time: 5 min

Icons: 🌱 Plant-Based option ⏱ Under 30 Min

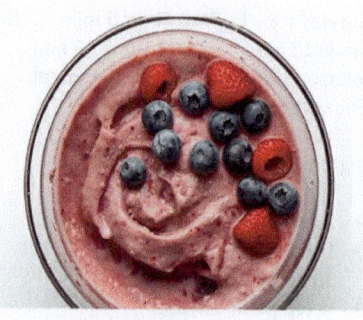

## Ingredients

- 1 cup low-fat cottage cheese
- 1 scoop vanilla protein powder
- ½ cup frozen mixed berries
- 1 tsp honey (optional)

## Directions

1. Blend cottage cheese, protein powder, berries, and honey until fluffy.
2. Chill before serving if desired.

## Nutrition (per serving)

- Calories: 180
- Protein: 22 g
- Carbs: 14 g (Fiber: 3 g)
- Fat: 3 g

## Storage & Prep

- Refrigerate up to 2 days.
- Not freezer-friendly.

# Chapter 12

# 50+ & Active Aging Meals

✦

Nutrition needs evolve as we age, and a high-protein diet can be one of the most powerful tools for maintaining strength, independence, and energy. For those 50 and beyond, protein helps preserve lean muscle, support bone health, and keep metabolism steady. But it's not just about the grams—you also need meals that are **easy to chew, nutrient-dense, and rich in calcium, vitamin D, and omega-3s** to protect both bone and heart health.

In this chapter, you'll find 10 recipes crafted specifically for active aging. They're designed to be gentle on digestion and teeth, while delivering big benefits in smaller, satisfying portions. From **soft-textured fish dishes rich in omega-3s** to **creamy soups and stews packed with calcium and protein**, each meal is practical, flavorful, and tailored to the nutritional priorities of this stage of life.

These recipes prove that eating for longevity doesn't mean sacrificing taste. They're simple to prepare, easy to enjoy, and built to help you stay strong, active, and vibrant well into your 50s, 60s, and beyond.

# Recipe Icons Guide

🔍 **One-Pan**
Cook the whole meal in a single pan —
less cleanup, more convenience.

❄️ **Freezer-Friendly**
Can be stored in the freezer for later;
reheats well.

$ **Budget-Friendly**
Costs under $4 per serving with
common ingredients.

⏱️ **Under 30 Minutes**
From prep to plate in half an hour or
less.

⭐ **30+ g Protein**
Each serving delivers at least 30 grams
of protein.

🌱 **Plant-Based**
Fully vegetarian or vegan protein
sources.

# Creamy Salmon & Spinach Skillet

Servings: 2 | Prep Time: 10 min | Cook Time: 15 min | Total Time: 25 min
Icons: $ Budget-Friendly 🔍 One-Pan ⏱ Under 30 Min

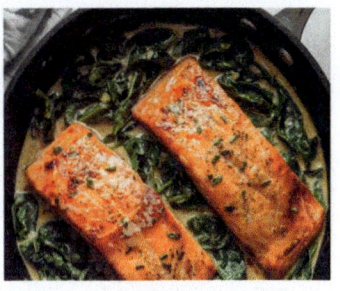

## Ingredients

- 2 salmon fillets (6 oz each)
- 1 tbsp olive oil
- 1 cup spinach
- ½ cup low-fat Greek yogurt
- Juice of ½ lemon
- 1 tsp dill

## Directions

1. Heat oil in skillet; cook salmon 4–5 minutes per side until flaky.
2. Remove salmon and stir spinach, yogurt, lemon juice, and dill into pan.
3. Return salmon to skillet and coat with sauce.

Nutrition (per serving)

- Calories: 330
- Protein: 36 g
- Carbs: 6 g
- Fat: 18 g (rich in omega-3s)

Storage & Prep

- Refrigerate up to 3 days.
- Not freezer-friendly.

# Soft Turkey & Vegetable Shepherd's Pie

Servings: 4 | Prep Time: 20 min | Cook Time: 30 min | Total Time: 50 min
Icons: $ Budget-Friendly ❄ Freezer-Friendly

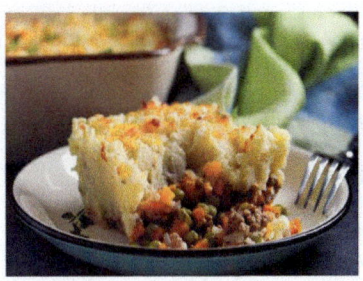

## Ingredients

- 1 lb ground turkey
- 1 onion, diced
- 2 carrots, diced
- 1 cup peas
- 2 tbsp tomato paste
- 4 cups mashed potatoes (made with milk + a little butter)

## Directions

1. Brown turkey with onion and carrots. Stir in peas and tomato paste.
2. Spread into casserole dish.
3. Top with mashed potatoes; bake 25–30 minutes at 375°F (190°C).

Nutrition (per serving)

- Calories: 380
- Protein: 30 g
- Carbs: 40 g (Fiber: 6 g)
- Fat: 11 g

Storage & Prep

- Refrigerate up to 4 days.
- Freeze up to 2 months.

# Creamy Sardine & Avocado Toast

Servings: 2  |  Prep Time: 5 min  |  Total Time: 5 min
Icons: 🌱 Plant-Based option  ⏱ Under 30 Min  $ Budget-Friendly

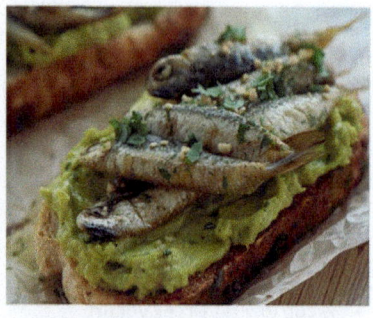

## Ingredients

- 1 can (3.75 oz) sardines in olive oil, drained
- 1 ripe avocado
- 2 slices whole grain bread, toasted
- Juice of ½ lemon
- Salt & pepper, to taste

## Directions

1. Mash avocado with lemon juice, salt, and pepper.
2. Spread on toast and top with sardines.

## Nutrition (per serving)

- Calories: 310
- Protein: 20 g
- Carbs: 22 g (Fiber: 6 g)
- Fat: 17 g (rich in omega-3s)

## Storage & Prep

- Best eaten fresh.
- Not freezer-friendly.

# High-Protein Creamy Broccoli Soup

Servings: 4  |  Prep Time: 10 min  |  Cook Time: 20 min  |  Total Time: 30 min
Icons: 🌱 Plant-Based option  🍲 One-Pot  ❄ Freezer-Friendly

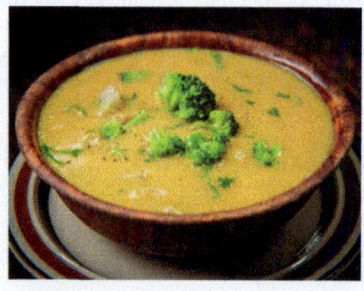

## Ingredients

- 3 cups broccoli florets
- 1 onion, diced
- 2 cups low-sodium chicken or veggie broth
- 1 cup low-fat milk
- 1 cup cottage cheese
- 1 tbsp olive oil

## Directions

1. Heat oil; sauté onion until soft.
2. Add broccoli and broth; simmer 10 minutes.
3. Blend with milk and cottage cheese until smooth.

## Nutrition (per serving)

- Calories: 220
- Protein: 18 g
- Carbs: 17 g (Fiber: 5 g)
- Fat: 8 g

## Storage & Prep

- Refrigerate up to 4 days.
- Freeze up to 2 months.

# Baked Cod with Sweet Potato Mash

Servings: 2  |  Prep Time: 10 min  |  Cook
Time: 25 min  |  Total Time: 35 min
Icons: $ Budget-Friendly  ❄ Freezer-
Friendly

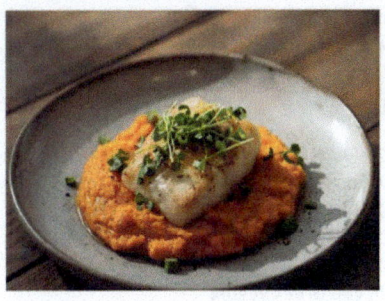

## Ingredients

- 2 cod fillets (6 oz each)
- 2 medium sweet potatoes, peeled and
  cubed
- 1 tbsp olive oil
- 1 tsp paprika
- Salt & pepper, to taste

## Directions

1. Boil sweet potatoes until tender; mash
   with olive oil, salt, and pepper.
2. Bake cod at 375°F (190°C) for 15–20
   minutes, seasoned with paprika.
3. Serve cod over sweet potato mash.

Nutrition (per serving)

- Calories: 320
- Protein: 34 g
- Carbs: 28 g (Fiber: 5 g)
- Fat: 8 g

Storage & Prep

- Refrigerate up to 3 days.
- Freeze fillets and mash separately up to 2 months.

# Baked Lemon Herb Trout

Servings: 2  |  Prep Time: 5 min  |  Cook
Time: 15 min  |  Total Time: 20 min
Icons: $ Budget-Friendly  ❄ Freezer-
Friendly

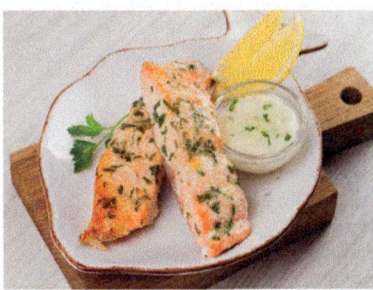

## Ingredients

- 2 trout fillets (6 oz each)
- 1 tbsp olive oil
- 1 tsp dried parsley
- ½ tsp garlic powder
- Juice of ½ lemon

## Directions

1. Preheat oven to 375°F (190°C).
2. Place trout on lined baking sheet; drizzle
   with oil, parsley, garlic, and lemon juice.
3. Bake 12–15 minutes until fish flakes
   easily.

Nutrition (per serving)

- Calories: 280
- Protein: 32 g
- Carbs: 1 g
- Fat: 16 g (rich in omega-3s)

Storage & Prep

- Refrigerate up to 3 days.
- Freeze fillets up to 2 months.

# Creamy White Bean & Kale Stew

Servings: 4 | Prep Time: 10 min | Cook Time: 25 min | Total Time: 35 min
Icons: 🌱 Plant-Based 🍲 One-Pot ❄️ Freezer-Friendly

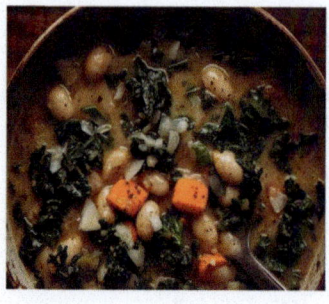

## Ingredients

- 2 cans (15 oz each) white beans, rinsed
- 4 cups low-sodium vegetable broth
- 2 cups kale, chopped
- 1 onion, diced
- 1 cup diced carrots
- ½ cup Greek yogurt
- 1 tsp thyme

## Nutrition (per serving)

- Calories: 260
- Protein: 20 g
- Carbs: 34 g (Fiber: 9 g)
- Fat: 6 g

## Directions

1. Sauté onion and carrots until soft.
2. Add beans, broth, kale, and thyme. Simmer 20 minutes.
3. Stir in yogurt before serving for creaminess.

## Storage & Prep

- Refrigerate up to 4 days.
- Freeze up to 2 months.

# Soft Baked Eggplant Parmesan

Servings: 4 | Prep Time: 15 min | Cook Time: 30 min | Total Time: 45 min
Icons: 🌱 Plant-Based 💲 Budget-Friendly ❄️ Freezer-Friendly

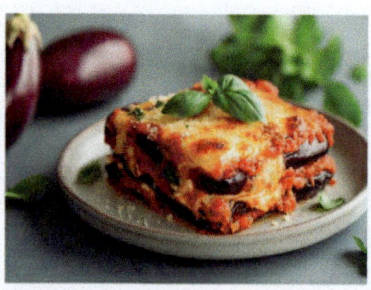

## Ingredients

- 2 medium eggplants, sliced into rounds
- 1 cup breadcrumbs (or almond flour)
- 2 eggs, beaten
- 2 cups marinara sauce
- 1 cup shredded mozzarella
- ½ cup grated Parmesan

## Nutrition (per serving)

- Calories: 310
- Protein: 22 g
- Carbs: 28 g (Fiber: 6 g)
- Fat: 12 g

## Directions

1. Preheat oven to 375°F (190°C).
2. Dip eggplant slices in egg, then breadcrumbs. Arrange in baking dish.
3. Top with marinara, mozzarella, and Parmesan.
4. Bake 25–30 minutes until tender and bubbly.

## Storage & Prep

- Refrigerate up to 3 days.
- Freeze portions up to 2 months.

# High-Protein Tuna & White Bean Salad

Servings: 3  |  Prep Time: 10 min  |  Total
Time: 10 min
Icons: $ Budget-Friendly  ⏱ Under 30 Min

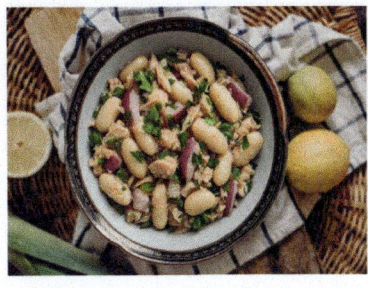

## Ingredients

- 2 cans (5 oz each) tuna, drained
- 1 can (15 oz) white beans, rinsed
- 2 tbsp olive oil
- 1 tbsp lemon juice
- 1 tbsp parsley, chopped

## Directions

1. Mix tuna, beans, olive oil, lemon juice, and parsley.
2. Chill before serving.

### Nutrition (per serving)

- Calories: 260
- Protein: 27 g
- Carbs: 14 g (Fiber: 5 g)
- Fat: 9 g

### Storage & Prep

- Refrigerate up to 3 days.
- Not freezer-friendly.

# Creamy Chia Seed Pudding with Almonds

Servings: 2  |  Prep Time: 5 min  |  Chill
Time: 4 hrs  |  Total Time: 4 hrs+
Icons: 🌱 Plant-Based  ❄ Freezer-Friendly

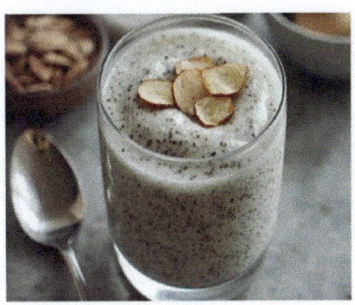

## Ingredients

- ¼ cup chia seeds
- 1 cup fortified almond milk (with calcium + vitamin D)
- 1 scoop vanilla protein powder
- 2 tbsp sliced almonds
- ½ tsp cinnamon

## Directions

1. Mix chia seeds, almond milk, protein powder, and cinnamon.
2. Stir well; refrigerate 4 hours or overnight.
3. Top with almonds before serving.

### Nutrition (per serving)

- Calories: 230
- Protein: 19 g
- Carbs: 18 g (Fiber: 8 g)
- Fat: 9 g

### Storage & Prep

- Refrigerate up to 5 days.
- Freeze in jars up to 1 month.

# Part
# IV
# Meal Plans & Tools

# Chapter 13

# 30-Day High-Protein Meal Plan

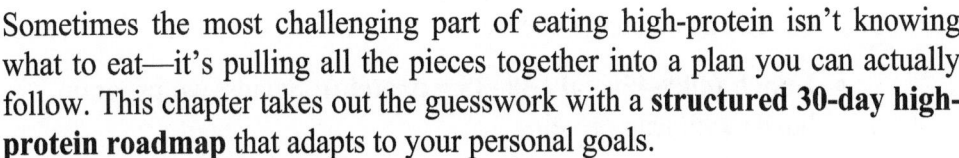

Sometimes the most challenging part of eating high-protein isn't knowing what to eat—it's pulling all the pieces together into a plan you can actually follow. This chapter takes out the guesswork with a **structured 30-day high-protein roadmap** that adapts to your personal goals.

You'll find two complete tracks:

- **Weight Loss Track** – Portion-controlled, calorie-conscious meals that keep protein high for satiety, lean muscle retention, and steady energy.

- **Muscle Gain Track** – Slightly higher calorie meals with balanced carbs and healthy fats to support recovery, training, and muscle growth.

Each track includes **weekly grocery lists, prep timelines,** and **freezer notes** so you'll always know what to shop, prep, and store. You'll also see how to **batch-cook base proteins and sides** to cut down on time while still enjoying variety.

This 30-day plan is designed to feel practical and flexible—not rigid. It will help you build consistency, reduce decision fatigue, and prove that with the right system, eating high-protein is both achievable and sustainable.

## Weekly Structure Overview

## Weight Loss Track

- **Goal:** Preserve lean muscle while creating a gentle calorie deficit.

- **Daily Protein Target:** ~100–130 g protein
- **Calories per Day:** ~1,500–1,800 (adjustable)

## Structure per Day

- **Breakfast (300–350 cal / 25–30 g protein):** High-protein oats, egg scrambles, yogurt bowls.
- **Snack (150–200 cal / 10–15 g protein):** Protein smoothies, boiled eggs, cottage cheese.
- **Lunch (400–450 cal / 30–35 g protein):** Salads, wraps, grain bowls with lean protein.
- **Snack (150–200 cal / 10–15 g protein):** Protein balls, edamame, tuna cucumber bites.
- **Dinner (450–500 cal / 35–40 g protein):** Simple sheet-pan meals, soups, lean meat or fish with veggies.

## Prep Focus

- Bulk-prep proteins (chicken, turkey, lentils, eggs).
- Freeze-ready portions for quick lunches/dinners.
- Emphasis on lighter but filling meals with fiber.

## Muscle Gain Track

- **Goal:** Support muscle growth and recovery with a slight calorie surplus.
- **Daily Protein Target:** ~140–160 g protein
- **Calories per Day:** ~2,200–2,500 (adjustable)

## Structure per Day

- **Breakfast (400–500 cal / 30–35 g protein):** Protein pancakes, smoothies with oats + protein powder, omelets with cheese.

- **Snack (200–250 cal / 15–20 g protein):** Cottage cheese bowls, nut butter + protein shakes.

- **Lunch (500–600 cal / 35–40 g protein):** Larger portions of rice bowls, wraps, chili, or stir-fries.

- **Snack (200–300 cal / 15–20 g protein):** Protein bars, yogurt parfaits, trail mix with added protein.

- **Dinner (600–700 cal / 40–45 g protein):** Balanced meals with lean protein, complex carbs, and healthy fats (e.g., salmon with rice and avocado, turkey pasta bake).

## Prep Focus

- Double portions of base proteins (chicken, salmon, lentils, eggs).

- Larger carb bases (rice, quinoa, potatoes) prepped in bulk.

- More calorie-dense snack options to hit surplus without excessive volume.

☑ Each week in both tracks includes:

- **Grocery list (grouped by protein, produce, pantry, freezer)**

- **Prep timeline (batch proteins, cooked grains, ready-to-eat snacks)**

- **Freezer notes (what to prep ahead, what freezes best)**

# Week 1: High-Protein Meal Plan

## Week 1 Grocery List (for 2 people)

### Proteins

- Chicken breast (6–8 lbs)
- Salmon fillets (4–6 fillets)
- Ground turkey (2 lbs)
- Eggs (2 dozen)
- Greek yogurt (2 large tubs, plain)
- Cottage cheese (2 tubs)
- Tuna (4 cans)
- Whey or plant protein powder (1 tub)

### Pantry

- Quinoa (2 lbs)
- Brown rice (2 lbs)
- Rolled oats (2 lbs)
- Chickpeas (4 cans or dry equivalent)
- Black beans/lentils (6 cans or dry equivalent)
- Whole wheat pasta/pita (1 pack each)
- Olive oil, soy sauce, spices (paprika, garlic, cumin, chili powder, cinnamon)

## Produce

- Spinach (2 bags)
- Broccoli (3–4 heads)
- Sweet potatoes (5–6 medium)
- Carrots (2 lbs)
- Bell peppers (3–4)
- Onions (3–4)
- Zucchini (2–3)
- Bananas (6)
- Berries, frozen (2 lbs)
- Lemons (2–3)

## Extras

- Peanut butter/almond butter
- Granola or trail mix
- Protein bars (optional, for muscle gain track)

# Prep Guide (Week 1)

**Day Before (Sunday)**

- Cook **quinoa (4 cups dry)** for bowls.
- Roast or bake **chicken breast (4 lbs)**, cube for salads + lunches.
- Make **overnight oats (5 jars)** for breakfasts.
- Chop veggies (carrots, peppers, cucumbers) for snacks.
- Hard-boil **12 eggs** for snacks.

## Midweek (Wednesday)

- Bake another batch of **sheet-pan salmon or chicken** for dinners.

- Cook **2 cups of rice** for sides.

- Prepare **meatballs or chili** (store half in freezer).

## Freezer Notes

- Freeze extra meatballs, chili, and cooked chicken in portion sizes.

- Overnight oats and smoothies can be prepped as freezer packs (fruit + powder in bags).

☑ This structure makes **Week 1 flexible:** batch proteins, mix-and-match lunches/dinners, snack variety, and freezer backup.

# Daily Menus: Side-by-Side (Week 1: Days 1-7)

## Day 1

**Weight Loss Track (~1,650 cal / 120 g protein)**

- Breakfast: Greek yogurt + protein powder + berries + chia (28 g protein)
- Snack: 2 boiled eggs + cucumber sticks (14 g protein)
- Lunch: Chicken & quinoa salad with spinach + vinaigrette (32 g protein)
- Snack: Roasted chickpeas (12 g protein)
- Dinner: Sheet-pan salmon with broccoli + sweet potato (34 g protein)

**Muscle Gain Track (~2,350 cal / 150 g protein)**

- Breakfast: Protein smoothie (milk, banana, oats, protein powder, PB) (32 g protein)
- Snack: Cottage cheese + granola + almonds (20 g protein)
- Lunch: Chicken & quinoa power bowl with avocado + chickpeas (38 g protein)
- Snack: Trail mix + protein bar (22 g protein)
- Dinner: Sheet-pan salmon with broccoli + sweet potato + rice (38 g protein)

## Day 2

**Weight Loss Track (~1,700 cal / 120 g protein)**

- Breakfast: Overnight oats with whey protein + PB (27 g protein / ~350 cal)
- Snack: Edamame with sea salt (15 g protein / ~180 cal)
- Lunch: Lentil & turkey soup (30 g protein / ~400 cal)
- Snack: Greek yogurt ranch dip + carrots (12 g protein / ~150 cal)
- Dinner: Garlic butter chicken & broccoli skillet (36 g protein / ~600 cal)

**Muscle Gain Track (~2,400 cal / 156 g protein)**

- Breakfast: Protein pancakes with cottage cheese topping (34 g protein / ~450 cal)
- Snack: Edamame + almonds (20 g protein / ~250 cal)
- Lunch: Lentil & turkey soup with added quinoa (38 g protein / ~550 cal)
- Snack: Greek yogurt + protein powder + granola (24 g protein / ~300 cal)
- Dinner: Garlic butter chicken & broccoli skillet + roasted potatoes (40 g protein / ~850 cal)

Weight Loss Track (~1,650 cal / 123 g protein)

- Breakfast: Scrambled eggs + spinach + toast (26 g protein / ~320 cal)
- Snack: Protein smoothie (Greek yogurt + berries) (18 g protein / ~200 cal)
- Lunch: Tuna & white bean salad (32 g protein / ~400 cal)
- Snack: Cottage cheese + pineapple (13 g protein / ~150 cal)
- Dinner: Turkey meatballs with zucchini noodles + marinara (34 g protein / ~580 cal)

Muscle Gain Track (~2,350 cal / 160 g protein)

- Breakfast: Protein oats (milk, oats, protein powder, PB) (32 g protein / ~450 cal)
- Snack: Protein smoothie (Greek yogurt, protein powder, banana, oats) (26 g protein / ~320 cal)
- Lunch: Tuna & white bean salad + whole wheat pita (38 g protein / ~500 cal)
- Snack: Cottage cheese + trail mix (20 g protein / ~250 cal)
- Dinner: Turkey meatballs with whole wheat pasta + marinara (42 g protein / ~830 cal)

# Day 4

Weight Loss Track (~1,650 cal / 122 g protein)

- Breakfast: Protein mug cake (90 seconds) with berries (26 g protein)
- Snack: Cottage cheese + sliced cucumber (14 g protein)
- Lunch: Turkey & avocado lettuce wraps (30 g protein)
- Snack: Protein balls (peanut butter + oats + protein powder) (12 g protein)
- Dinner: Slow cooker pulled BBQ chicken + broccoli slaw (40 g protein)

Muscle Gain Track (~2,350 cal / 154 g protein)

- Breakfast: Protein mug cake with PB drizzle + banana (32 g protein)
- Snack: Cottage cheese + granola + almonds (20 g protein)
- Lunch: Turkey & avocado wraps with quinoa side (38 g protein)
- Snack: Protein smoothie (milk, protein powder, oats, banana) (24 g protein)
- Dinner: Pulled BBQ chicken + slaw + roasted sweet potatoes (40 g protein)

**Weight Loss Track (~1,700 cal / 125 g protein)**

- Breakfast: Scrambled eggs + spinach + feta (28 g protein)
- Snack: Greek yogurt + chia + blueberries (18 g protein)
- Lunch: Lentil & quinoa Buddha bowl with roasted veggies (32 g protein)
- Snack: Edamame with sea salt (14 g protein)
- Dinner: Garlic butter shrimp stir-fry with zucchini noodles (33 g protein)

**Muscle Gain Track (~2,400 cal / 156 g protein)**

- Breakfast: Scrambled eggs + spinach + feta + 2 slices toast (32 g protein)
- Snack: Greek yogurt + protein powder + oats + blueberries (24 g protein)
- Lunch: Lentil & quinoa Buddha bowl with added chicken breast (40 g protein)
- Snack: Edamame + almonds (20 g protein)
- Dinner: Garlic butter shrimp stir-fry with zucchini noodles + brown rice (40 g protein)

## Day 6

**Weight Loss Track (~1,650 cal / 120 g protein)**

- Breakfast: Cottage cheese + pineapple + walnuts (24 g protein)
- Snack: Protein smoothie (milk + protein powder + banana) (22 g protein)
- Lunch: Tuna & avocado cucumber roll-ups (30 g protein)
- Snack: Roasted chickpeas (12 g protein)
- Dinner: One-pot beef & lentil chili (32 g protein)

**Muscle Gain Track (~2,350 cal / 152 g protein)**

- Breakfast: Cottage cheese + pineapple + walnuts + granola (28 g protein)
- Snack: Protein smoothie (milk + protein powder + oats + PB) (28 g protein)
- Lunch: Tuna & avocado wraps + quinoa salad (38 g protein)
- Snack: Roasted chickpeas + Greek yogurt (22 g protein)
- Dinner: One-pot beef & lentil chili with whole wheat bread (36 g protein)

**Weight Loss Track (~1,700 cal / 123 g protein)**

- Breakfast: High-protein smoothie (milk, protein powder, berries, spinach) (30 g protein)
- Snack: Boiled eggs (2) + carrot sticks (14 g protein)
- Lunch: Greek chickpea salad with feta (veg) (28 g protein)
- Snack: Cottage cheese + strawberries (13 g protein)
- Dinner: Sheet-pan chicken & veggies with quinoa (38 g protein)

**Muscle Gain Track (~2,400 cal / 158 g protein)**

- Breakfast: High-protein smoothie with oats + PB added (36 g protein)
- Snack: Boiled eggs (3) + whole grain toast (20 g protein)
- Lunch: Greek chickpea salad + grilled chicken (36 g protein)
- Snack: Cottage cheese parfait with granola + almonds (26 g protein)
- Dinner: Sheet-pan chicken & veggies with quinoa + roasted potatoes (40 g protein)

# Week 2: High-Protein Meal Plan

## Week 2 Grocery List

(for 2 people, both tracks combined — scale up/down as needed)

## Proteins

- Chicken breast (6–8 lbs)
- Ground turkey (2 lbs)
- Salmon fillets (4–6 fillets)
- White fish (cod/tilapia, 4–6 fillets)
- Lean ground beef (1 lb)
- Eggs (2 dozen)
- Greek yogurt (2 large tubs)
- Cottage cheese (2 tubs)
- Whey or plant protein powder (1 tub)
- Tuna (4 cans)
- Edamame (frozen, 2 lbs)
- Black beans (3 cans)
- Lentils (3 cups dry or 3 cans)

## Grains & Pantry

- Brown rice (2 lbs)
- Quinoa (2 lbs)
- Rolled oats (2 lbs)

- Whole wheat wraps (1 pack)
- Whole wheat pasta (1 lb)
- Chickpeas (4 cans)
- Peanut butter/almond butter
- Olive oil, sesame oil
- Spices: chili powder, cumin, garlic powder, paprika, Italian seasoning
- Soy sauce, low-sodium
- Tomato paste (2 small cans)
- Canned crushed tomatoes (2 large cans)

## Produce

- Spinach (2 bags)
- Broccoli (3–4 heads)
- Zucchini (3–4)
- Carrots (2 lbs)
- Bell peppers (4–5)
- Onions (4–5)
- Sweet potatoes (5–6)
- White potatoes (3–4)
- Cucumbers (3–4)
- Lemons (3)
- Bananas (6)
- Apples (4–6)

- Berries, frozen (2 lbs)
- Avocados (3–4)

## Extras

- Protein bars (optional, muscle gain)
- Granola or trail mix
- Almonds (1 bag)
- Low-fat shredded mozzarella or cheddar (1 bag)
- Whole grain bread (1 loaf)

# Week 2 Prep Guide

## Day Before (Sunday)

### Batch Proteins

- Bake/roast for **4 lbs chicken breasts** (cube for bowls, shred for wraps).
- Cook **1 lb. ground turkey** (use for stuffed peppers and wraps).
- Hard-boil **12 eggs** for snacks.

### Cook Grains

- Cook 4 **cups dry quinoa** (≈12 cups cooked).
- Cook **3 cups dry brown rice** (≈9 cups cooked).

### Prep Snacks

- Make a batch of protein balls (oats + PB + protein powder).
- Roast a tray of chickpeas (seasoned).

**Veg Prep**

- Chop carrots, peppers, and cucumbers for grab-and-go.
- Steam 4 cups of broccoli for sides/snacks.

# Midweek (Wednesday)

1. Bake 2–3 **salmon fillets** for quick dinners/lunches.

2. Cook **2 cups of pasta** for Buddha bowls + quick pasta dishes.

3. Assemble a **pot of chili or lentil soup** (half to fridge, half to freezer).

# Freezer Notes

- Freeze extra cooked proteins (chicken, turkey, salmon) in single-serve bags.
- Soup, chili, and meatballs freeze well up to 3 months.
- Overnight oats can be portioned into freezer jars (add fruit before serving).

✅ This keeps **Week 2 organized and stress-free.** You'll cook most of your proteins and grains once, then repurpose them into different lunches/dinners across the week for both tracks.

# Daily Menus: Side-by-Side (Week 2: Days 8-14)

## Day 8

**Weight Loss Track (~1,650 cal / 122 g protein)**

- Breakfast: Greek yogurt parfait with protein powder + berries + chia (28 g protein)
- Snack: 2 boiled eggs + cucumber slices (14 g protein)
- Lunch: Lentil & veggie soup with quinoa (30 g protein)
- Snack: Protein ball (oats + PB + protein powder) (12 g protein)
- Dinner: Garlic butter chicken with roasted broccoli + sweet potato (38 g protein)

**Muscle Gain Track (~2,350 cal / 154 g protein)**

- Breakfast: Protein oats with banana + PB drizzle (32 g protein)
- Snack: Cottage cheese with granola + almonds (20 g protein)
- Lunch: Lentil & veggie soup with quinoa + shredded chicken (40 g protein)
- Snack: Protein smoothie (milk, protein powder, oats, banana) (24 g protein)
- Dinner: Garlic butter chicken with broccoli, sweet potato + rice (38 g protein)

## Day 9

**Weight Loss Track (~1,700 cal / 124 g protein)**

- Breakfast: Scrambled eggs + spinach + whole wheat toast (28 g protein)
- Snack: Greek yogurt with chia + berries (18 g protein)
- Lunch: Tuna & avocado cucumber roll-ups (30 g protein)
- Snack: Roasted chickpeas (12 g protein)
- Dinner: Beef & lentil chili (36 g protein)

**Muscle Gain Track (~2,400 cal / 156 g protein)**

- Breakfast: Protein smoothie (milk, oats, banana, protein powder, PB) (34 g protein)
- Snack: Greek yogurt + protein powder + granola (24 g protein)
- Lunch: Tuna & avocado wraps + quinoa side (38 g protein)
- Snack: Cottage cheese + almonds (20 g protein)
- Dinner: Beef & lentil chili with whole wheat bread (40 g protein)

# Day 10

**Weight Loss Track (~1,650 cal / 120 g protein)**

- Breakfast: Overnight oats with protein powder + berries (27 g protein)
- Snack: Cottage cheese with apple slices (14 g protein)
- Lunch: Turkey & quinoa stuffed peppers (30 g protein)
- Snack: Edamame with sea salt (15 g protein)
- Dinner: Sheet-pan salmon with zucchini + carrots (34 g protein)

**Muscle Gain Track (~2,350 cal / 152 g protein)**

- Breakfast: Overnight oats with protein powder, banana + PB (32 g protein)
- Snack: Cottage cheese + granola + almonds (20 g protein)
- Lunch: Turkey & quinoa stuffed peppers with extra rice (38 g protein)
- Snack: Protein smoothie (milk, protein powder, oats) (26 g protein)
- Dinner: Sheet-pan salmon with zucchini, carrots + brown rice (36 g protein)

# Day 11

**Weight Loss Track (~1,700 cal / 125 g protein)**

- Breakfast: Protein pancakes with Greek yogurt topping (28 g protein)
- Snack: 2 boiled eggs + carrots (14 g protein)
- Lunch: Black bean & quinoa salad with lime dressing (28 g protein)
- Snack: Cottage cheese + pineapple (13 g protein)
- Dinner: Chicken stir-fry with broccoli + peppers (42 g protein)

**Muscle Gain Track (~2,400 cal / 158 g protein)**

- Breakfast: Protein pancakes topped with yogurt + PB drizzle (34 g protein)
- Snack: Cottage cheese + almonds (20 g protein)
- Lunch: Black bean & quinoa salad + shredded chicken (38 g protein)
- Snack: Protein smoothie (milk, protein powder, oats, banana) (24 g protein)
- Dinner: Chicken stir-fry with broccoli, peppers + rice (42 g protein)

**Weight Loss Track (~1,650 cal / 121 g protein)**

- Breakfast: Greek yogurt with chia seeds + strawberries (26 g protein)
- Snack: Protein smoothie (Greek yogurt + protein powder + berries) (20 g protein)
- Lunch: Tuna & white bean salad (30 g protein)
- Snack: Edamame (14 g protein)
- Dinner: Baked cod with mashed sweet potato + spinach (31 g protein)

**Muscle Gain Track (~2,350 cal / 153 g protein)**

- Breakfast: Protein smoothie with oats, PB, banana, protein powder (34 g protein)
- Snack: Greek yogurt + granola + protein powder (24 g protein)
- Lunch: Tuna & white bean salad + whole wheat pita (38 g protein)
- Snack: Cottage cheese + almonds (20 g protein)
- Dinner: Baked cod with mashed sweet potato, spinach + rice (37 g protein)

# Day 13

**Weight Loss Track (~1,700 cal / 124 g protein)**

- Breakfast: Scrambled eggs + spinach + feta (28 g protein)
- Snack: Cottage cheese with cucumber slices (14 g protein)
- Lunch: Chickpea & veggie power bowl with tahini dressing (28 g protein)
- Snack: Protein balls (12 g protein)
- Dinner: Slow cooker turkey chili with beans (42 g protein)

**Muscle Gain Track (~2,400 cal / 156 g protein)**

- Breakfast: Scrambled eggs + spinach + feta + toast (32 g protein)
- Snack: Greek yogurt + protein powder + oats (24 g protein)
- Lunch: Chickpea & veggie power bowl + grilled chicken (38 g protein)
- Snack: Protein smoothie (milk, protein powder, banana, oats) (24 g protein)
- Dinner: Slow cooker turkey chili with beans + rice (38 g protein)

**Weight Loss Track (~1,650 cal / 122 g protein)**

- Breakfast: Protein mug cake with banana slices (28 g protein)
- Snack: Boiled eggs (2) + carrots (14 g protein)
- Lunch: Turkey & avocado lettuce wraps (30 g protein)
- Snack: Roasted chickpeas (12 g protein)
- Dinner: Garlic butter shrimp with zucchini noodles (38 g protein)

**Muscle Gain Track (~2,350 cal / 154 g protein)**

- Breakfast: Protein mug cake with PB + oats mixed in (34 g protein)
- Snack: Cottage cheese + granola (20 g protein)
- Lunch: Turkey & avocado wraps + quinoa salad (38 g protein)
- Snack: Protein smoothie (milk, protein powder, oats, banana) (24 g protein)
- Dinner: Garlic butter shrimp with zucchini noodles + rice (38 g protein)

# Week 3: High-Protein Meal Plan

## Week 3 Grocery List

(for 2 people, both tracks combined — scale as needed)

## Proteins

- Chicken breast (6–8 lbs)
- Ground turkey (2 lbs)
- Salmon fillets (4–6 fillets)
- White fish (cod or tilapia, 4 fillets)
- Lean ground beef (1 lb)
- Eggs (2 dozen)
- Greek yogurt (2 large tubs)
- Cottage cheese (2 tubs)
- Whey or plant protein powder (1 tub)
- Tuna (4 cans)
- Shrimp (2 lbs)
- Black beans (3 cans)
- Lentils (3 cups dry or 3 cans)

## Grains & Pantry

- Quinoa (2 lbs)
- Brown rice (2 lbs)
- Rolled oats (2 lbs)

- Whole wheat wraps (1 pack)
- Whole grain bread (1 loaf)
- Chickpeas (4 cans)
- Peanut butter/almond butter
- Olive oil, sesame oil
- Spices: cumin, paprika, chili powder, Italian seasoning, turmeric
- Soy sauce (low sodium)
- Tomato paste (2 cans)
- Crushed tomatoes (2 cans)

## Produce

- Spinach (2 bags)
- Kale (1 bag)
- Broccoli (3–4 heads)
- Zucchini (3–4)
- Carrots (2 lbs)
- Bell peppers (4–5)
- Onions (4–5)
- Sweet potatoes (5–6)
- White potatoes (3–4)
- Cucumbers (3–4)
- Lemons (3)
- Bananas (6)
- Apples (4–6)

- Frozen berries (2 lbs)

- Avocados (3–4)

## Extras

- Almonds or walnuts (1 bag)

- Granola or trail mix

- Protein bars (optional for muscle gain)

- Low-fat shredded mozzarella or cheddar (1 bag)

# Week 3 Prep Guide

# Day Before (Sunday)

### Batch Proteins

- Cook **4 lbs chicken breast** (grilled, baked, or shredded).

- Brown **1 lb. lean ground beef** (use for chili or wraps).

- Boil **12 eggs** for snacks.

### Cook Grains

- Make **4 cups of dry quinoa** (≈12 cups cooked).

- Cook **3 cups dry brown rice** (≈9 cups cooked).

### Prep Snacks

- Make 8–10 protein balls (oats + PB + protein powder).

- Roast 2 cups of chickpeas with seasoning.

### Veg Prep

- Chop cucumbers, peppers, and carrots into snack sticks.

- Steam 4 cups of broccoli for quick sides.

# Midweek (Wednesday)

1. Bake **salmon fillets (3–4)** for quick dinners or lunches.

2. Cook **shrimp** (sauté or boil) for bowls and wraps.

3. Prepare a **large pot of lentil stew or bean chili** (half for fridge, half to freezer).

# Freezer Notes

- Freeze extra cooked proteins (chicken, salmon, shrimp) in meal-sized bags.

- Chili, stews, and soups freeze well up to 3 months.

- Protein pancakes or waffles can be batch-made and frozen, then reheated.

✅ Week 3 prep ensures variety with **shrimp, lentils, and stews** added into the rotation while still relying on batch proteins and grain bases.

# Day 15

**Weight Loss Track (~1,700 cal / 123 g protein)**

- Breakfast: Greek yogurt + protein powder + berries + chia (28 g protein / ~350 cal)
- Snack: Boiled eggs (2) + cucumber sticks (14 g protein / ~180 cal)
- Lunch: Chicken & lentil stew (30 g protein / ~400 cal)
- Snack: Roasted chickpeas (12 g protein / ~150 cal)
- Dinner: Shrimp stir-fry with broccoli + brown rice (39 g protein / ~620 cal)

**Muscle Gain Track (~2,400 cal / 158 g protein)**

- Breakfast: Protein oats with banana + PB drizzle (32 g protein / ~450 cal)
- Snack: Cottage cheese + granola + almonds (20 g protein / ~280 cal)
- Lunch: Chicken & lentil stew + quinoa (38 g protein / ~520 cal)
- Snack: Protein smoothie (milk, protein powder, oats, banana) (26 g protein / ~330 cal)
- Dinner: Shrimp stir-fry with broccoli + brown rice + avocado (42 g protein / ~820 cal)

# Day 16

**Weight Loss Track (~1,650 cal / 120 g protein)**

- Breakfast: Scrambled eggs + spinach + feta (28 g protein / ~330 cal)
- Snack: Greek yogurt + blueberries (18 g protein / ~200 cal)
- Lunch: Tuna & white bean salad (32 g protein / ~400 cal)
- Snack: Cottage cheese + apple slices (13 g protein / ~150 cal)
- Dinner: Garlic butter chicken & veggies (29 g protein / ~570 cal)

**Muscle Gain Track (~2,350 cal / 155 g protein)**

- Breakfast: Protein smoothie (milk, protein powder, oats, banana, PB) (34 g protein / ~450 cal)
- Snack: Greek yogurt + granola + protein powder (24 g protein / ~300 cal)
- Lunch: Tuna & white bean salad + quinoa (38 g protein / ~500 cal)
- Snack: Cottage cheese + almonds (20 g protein / ~250 cal)
- Dinner: Garlic butter chicken & veggies + sweet potato (39 g protein / ~850 cal)

# Day 17

**Weight Loss Track (~1,700 cal / 125 g protein)**

- Breakfast: Protein pancakes + Greek yogurt topping (28 g protein / ~350 cal)
- Snack: Edamame (15 g protein / ~180 cal)
- Lunch: Turkey & veggie chili (32 g protein / ~420 cal)
- Snack: Protein ball (12 g protein / ~150 cal)
- Dinner: Baked salmon + quinoa + asparagus (38 g protein / ~600 cal)

**Muscle Gain Track (~2,400 cal / 160 g protein)**

- Breakfast: Protein pancakes with yogurt + PB drizzle (34 g protein / ~460 cal)
- Snack: Cottage cheese + granola (20 g protein / ~280 cal)
- Lunch: Turkey & veggie chili + rice (38 g protein / ~500 cal)
- Snack: Protein smoothie (milk, protein powder, oats, banana) (26 g protein / ~330 cal)
- Dinner: Baked salmon + quinoa + asparagus + avocado (42 g protein / ~830 cal)

# Day 18

**Weight Loss Track (~1,650 cal / 122 g protein)**

- Breakfast: Overnight oats with protein powder + chia (27 g protein / ~350 cal)
- Snack: Cottage cheese + pineapple (14 g protein / ~150 cal)
- Lunch: Lentil & veggie soup (30 g protein / ~400 cal)
- Snack: Boiled eggs (2) + carrot sticks (14 g protein / ~180 cal)
- Dinner: Chicken stir-fry with broccoli + zucchini (37 g protein / ~570 cal)

**Muscle Gain Track (~2,350 cal / 157 g protein)**

- Breakfast: Overnight oats with protein powder + banana + PB (32 g protein / ~450 cal)
- Snack: Cottage cheese + granola + almonds (20 g protein / ~280 cal)
- Lunch: Lentil & veggie soup + shredded chicken (38 g protein / ~500 cal)
- Snack: Protein smoothie (milk, protein powder, oats, banana) (26 g protein / ~320 cal)
- Dinner: Chicken stir-fry with broccoli, zucchini + brown rice (41 g protein / ~800 cal)

**Weight Loss Track (~1,700 cal / 124 g protein)**

- Breakfast: Protein smoothie (Greek yogurt + berries + protein powder) (30 g protein / ~300 cal)
- Snack: Roasted chickpeas (12 g protein / ~150 cal)
- Lunch: Quinoa & black bean power bowl (28 g protein / ~400 cal)
- Snack: Greek yogurt + chia (14 g protein / ~200 cal)
- Dinner: Shrimp & veggie stir-fry (40 g protein / ~650 cal)

**Muscle Gain Track (~2,400 cal / 160 g protein)**

- Breakfast: Protein smoothie (milk, oats, PB, protein powder, banana) (36 g protein / ~450 cal)
- Snack: Cottage cheese + almonds (20 g protein / ~250 cal)
- Lunch: Quinoa & black bean power bowl + chicken (38 g protein / ~520 cal)
- Snack: Greek yogurt + granola + protein powder (26 g protein / ~300 cal)
- Dinner: Shrimp & veggie stir-fry + brown rice (40 g protein / ~880 cal)

# Day 20

**Weight Loss Track (~1,650 cal / 121 g protein)**

- Breakfast: Scrambled eggs + spinach + toast (26 g protein / ~320 cal)
- Snack: Edamame (15 g protein / ~180 cal)
- Lunch: Tuna & avocado cucumber rolls (30 g protein / ~400 cal)
- Snack: Protein ball (12 g protein / ~150 cal)
- Dinner: Turkey meatballs + zucchini noodles + marinara (38 g protein / ~600 cal)

**Muscle Gain Track (~2,350 cal / 156 g protein)**

- Breakfast: Protein oats (milk, oats, protein powder, PB) (32 g protein / ~450 cal)
- Snack: Edamame + almonds (20 g protein / ~250 cal)
- Lunch: Tuna & avocado wraps + quinoa salad (38 g protein / ~500 cal)
- Snack: Protein smoothie (milk, protein powder, oats, banana) (26 g protein / ~320 cal)
- Dinner: Turkey meatballs + whole wheat pasta + marinara (40 g protein / ~830 cal)

**Weight Loss Track (~1,700 cal / 123 g protein)**

- Breakfast: Greek yogurt + protein powder + banana (28 g protein / ~350 cal)
- Snack: Cottage cheese + cucumber slices (14 g protein / ~150 cal)
- Lunch: Chickpea & spinach Buddha bowl (30 g protein / ~420 cal)
- Snack: Protein ball (12 g protein / ~150 cal)
- Dinner: Garlic butter cod + mashed potatoes + broccoli (39 g protein / ~630 cal)

**Muscle Gain Track (~2,400 cal / 159 g protein)**

- Breakfast: Protein smoothie (milk, oats, banana, PB, protein powder) (34 g protein / ~450 cal)
- Snack: Cottage cheese + granola + almonds (20 g protein / ~280 cal)
- Lunch: Chickpea & spinach Buddha bowl + grilled chicken (38 g protein / ~500 cal)
- Snack: Greek yogurt + protein powder + granola (26 g protein / ~320 cal)
- Dinner: Garlic butter cod + mashed potatoes + broccoli + rice (41 g protein / ~850 cal)

# Week 4: High-Protein Meal Plan

## Week 4 Grocery List

(for 2 people, both tracks combined — scale as needed)

## Proteins

- Chicken breast (6–8 lbs)
- Ground turkey (2 lbs)
- Salmon fillets (4–6 fillets)
- Lean ground beef (1 lb)
- White fish (4 fillets, cod or tilapia)
- Shrimp (2 lbs)
- Eggs (2 dozen)
- Greek yogurt (2 large tubs)
- Cottage cheese (2 tubs)
- Whey or plant protein powder (1 tub)
- Tuna (4 cans)
- Lentils (3 cups dry or 3 cans)
- Chickpeas (4 cans)
- Edamame (frozen, 2 lbs)

## Grains & Pantry

- Brown rice (2 lbs)
- Quinoa (2 lbs)

- Rolled oats (2 lbs)
- Whole wheat wraps (1 pack)
- Whole grain bread (1 loaf)
- Whole wheat pasta (1 lb)
- Peanut butter/almond butter
- Olive oil, sesame oil
- Spices: chili powder, garlic powder, paprika, cumin, black pepper
- Soy sauce (low sodium)
- Tomato paste (2 small cans)
- Crushed tomatoes (2 large cans)

# Produce

- Spinach (2 bags)
- Broccoli (3–4 heads)
- Kale (1 bag)
- Zucchini (3–4)
- Carrots (2 lbs)
- Bell peppers (4–5)
- Onions (4–5)
- Sweet potatoes (5–6)
- White potatoes (3–4)
- Cucumbers (3–4)
- Lemons (3)
- Bananas (6)

- Apples (4–6)

- Frozen berries (2 lbs)

- Avocados (3–4)

## Extras

- Almonds or walnuts (1 bag)

- Granola or trail mix

- Protein bars (optional, for muscle gain)

- Low-fat shredded mozzarella or cheddar (1 bag)

- Greek feta or Parmesan (optional for salads/bowls)

# Week 4 Prep Guide

# Day Before (Sunday)

### Batch Proteins

- Grill or bake **4 lbs chicken breasts** (cube or shred).

- Cook **1 lb of ground turkey** for wraps and bowls.

- Hard-boil **12 eggs** for snacks.

### Cook Grains

- Prepare **4 cups of dry quinoa** (≈12 cups cooked).

- Cook **3 cups dry brown rice** (≈9 cups cooked).

- Make **2 cups of pasta** (for later meals).

### Prep Snacks

- Make a double batch of protein balls (oats + PB + protein powder).

- Roast 2 cups of chickpeas with olive oil and sea salt.

### Veg Prep

- Chop carrots, cucumbers, and peppers into snack-ready portions.

- Steam 4 cups of broccoli and store in containers for quick reheating.

# Midweek (Wednesday)

Bake **3–4 salmon fillets** and refrigerate for dinners and bowls.

Cook **shrimp or white fish** for quick proteins.

Make a **pot of turkey chili or lentil soup** (half to fridge, half to freezer).

# Freezer Notes

- Extra proteins (chicken, fish, shrimp) freeze up to 2 months.

- Chili, soups, and stews freeze up to 3 months.

- Cooked grains and roasted vegetables freeze well in single portions.

- Protein pancakes and mug cakes can be prepped and frozen for reheating.

✅ Week 4 continues the balance of **simplicity, prep efficiency, and variety** — with familiar core proteins and fresh combinations to finish out the 30-day plan strong.

# Daily Menus: Side-by-Side (Week 4: Days 22-28)

## Day 22

**Weight Loss Track (~1,650 cal / 121 g protein)**

- Breakfast: Scrambled eggs + spinach + toast (26 g protein / ~320 cal)
- Snack: Edamame (15 g protein / ~180 cal)
- Lunch: Tuna & avocado cucumber roll-ups (30 g protein / ~400 cal)
- Snack: Cottage cheese + pineapple (13 g protein / ~150 cal)
- Dinner: Turkey chili with beans (37 g protein / ~600 cal)

**Muscle Gain Track (~2,350 cal / 155 g protein)**

- Breakfast: Protein oats (milk, oats, protein powder, PB) (32 g protein / ~450 cal)
- Snack: Edamame + almonds (20 g protein / ~250 cal)
- Lunch: Tuna & avocado wraps + quinoa (38 g protein / ~500 cal)
- Snack: Cottage cheese + granola (20 g protein / ~250 cal)
- Dinner: Turkey chili with beans + brown rice (45 g protein / ~900 cal)

## Day 23

**Weight Loss Track (~1,700 cal / 122 g protein)**

- Breakfast: Greek yogurt + protein powder + banana (28 g protein / ~350 cal)
- Snack: Boiled eggs (2) + cucumber slices (14 g protein / ~180 cal)
- Lunch: Lentil & veggie soup (30 g protein / ~400 cal)
- Snack: Roasted chickpeas (12 g protein / ~150 cal)
- Dinner: Garlic butter salmon + broccoli + quinoa (38 g protein / ~620 cal)

**Muscle Gain Track (~2,400 cal / 158 g protein)**

- Breakfast: Protein smoothie (milk, oats, PB, protein powder, banana) (34 g protein / ~450 cal)
- Snack: Cottage cheese + granola + almonds (20 g protein / ~280 cal)
- Lunch: Lentil & veggie soup + shredded chicken (38 g protein / ~500 cal)
- Snack: Protein smoothie (milk, protein powder, banana) (24 g protein / ~330 cal)
- Dinner: Garlic butter salmon + broccoli + quinoa + sweet potato (42 g protein / ~850 cal)

# Day 24

**Weight Loss Track (~1,700 cal / 125 g protein)**

- Breakfast: Protein pancakes + Greek yogurt topping (28 g protein / ~350 cal)
- Snack: Greek yogurt + chia + berries (18 g protein / ~200 cal)
- Lunch: Chicken & quinoa salad with spinach + lemon vinaigrette (32 g protein / ~400 cal)
- Snack: Protein ball (12 g protein / ~150 cal)
- Dinner: Shrimp stir-fry with broccoli + zucchini noodles (35 g protein / ~600 cal)

**Muscle Gain Track (~2,400 cal / 160 g protein)**

- Breakfast: Protein pancakes with yogurt + PB drizzle (34 g protein / ~450 cal)
- Snack: Cottage cheese + granola + almonds (20 g protein / ~280 cal)
- Lunch: Chicken & quinoa salad with avocado + chickpeas (38 g protein / ~500 cal)
- Snack: Protein smoothie (milk, protein powder, oats, banana) (26 g protein / ~320 cal)
- Dinner: Shrimp stir-fry with broccoli, zucchini + brown rice (42 g protein / ~850 cal)

# Day 25

**Weight Loss Track (~1,650 cal / 120 g protein)**

- Breakfast: Overnight oats with protein powder + PB (27 g protein / ~350 cal)
- Snack: Boiled eggs (2) + carrots (14 g protein / ~180 cal)
- Lunch: Tuna & white bean salad (30 g protein / ~400 cal)
- Snack: Greek yogurt + chia (12 g protein / ~150 cal)
- Dinner: Garlic butter chicken + roasted veggies (37 g protein / ~570 cal)

**Muscle Gain Track (~2,350 cal / 156 g protein)**

- Breakfast: Protein oats (milk, oats, protein powder, PB) (32 g protein / ~450 cal)
- Snack: Cottage cheese + granola (20 g protein / ~250 cal)
- Lunch: Tuna & white bean salad + quinoa (38 g protein / ~500 cal)
- Snack: Protein smoothie (milk, protein powder, banana, oats) (26 g protein / ~320 cal)
- Dinner: Garlic butter chicken + roasted veggies + sweet potato (40 g protein / ~830 cal)

**Weight Loss Track (~1,700 cal / 124 g protein)**

- Breakfast: Greek yogurt + protein powder + berries (28 g protein / ~350 cal)
- Snack: Edamame (15 g protein / ~180 cal)
- Lunch: Lentil & quinoa bowl with veggies (32 g protein / ~400 cal)
- Snack: Protein ball (12 g protein / ~150 cal)
- Dinner: Baked cod + mashed potatoes + spinach (37 g protein / ~620 cal)

**Muscle Gain Track (~2,400 cal / 160 g protein)**

- Breakfast: Protein smoothie (milk, oats, PB, banana, protein powder) (34 g protein / ~450 cal)
- Snack: Cottage cheese + almonds (20 g protein / ~250 cal)
- Lunch: Lentil & quinoa bowl + grilled chicken (38 g protein / ~500 cal)
- Snack: Greek yogurt + protein powder + granola (28 g protein / ~320 cal)
- Dinner: Baked cod + mashed potatoes + spinach + brown rice (40 g protein / ~880 cal)

## Day 27

**Weight Loss Track (~1,650 cal / 121 g protein)**

- Breakfast: Scrambled eggs + spinach + feta (28 g protein / ~330 cal)
- Snack: Roasted chickpeas (12 g protein / ~150 cal)
- Lunch: Greek chickpea salad with feta (28 g protein / ~400 cal)
- Snack: Cottage cheese + apple slices (13 g protein / ~150 cal)
- Dinner: One-pot turkey & lentil chili (40 g protein / ~620 cal)

**Muscle Gain Track (~2,350 cal / 157 g protein)**

- Breakfast: Protein smoothie (milk, oats, PB, banana, protein powder) (34 g protein / ~450 cal)
- Snack: Cottage cheese + granola + almonds (20 g protein / ~280 cal)
- Lunch: Greek chickpea salad + grilled chicken (38 g protein / ~500 cal)
- Snack: Greek yogurt + protein powder + granola (25 g protein / ~300 cal)
- Dinner: Turkey & lentil chili + brown rice (40 g protein / ~820 cal)

**Weight Loss Track (~1,700 cal / 123 g protein)**

- Breakfast: Protein mug cake + banana slices (28 g protein / ~350 cal)
- Snack: Boiled eggs (2) + carrot sticks (14 g protein / ~180 cal)
- Lunch: Turkey & avocado lettuce wraps (30 g protein / ~400 cal)
- Snack: Greek yogurt + chia (12 g protein / ~150 cal)
- Dinner: Garlic butter shrimp + broccoli + sweet potato mash (39 g protein / ~620 cal)

**Muscle Gain Track (~2,400 cal / 159 g protein)**

- Breakfast: Protein mug cake with PB + oats mixed in (34 g protein / ~450 cal)
- Snack: Cottage cheese + granola + almonds (20 g protein / ~280 cal)
- Lunch: Turkey & avocado wraps + quinoa (38 g protein / ~500 cal)
- Snack: Protein smoothie (milk, protein powder, oats, banana) (26 g protein / ~320 cal)
- Dinner: Garlic butter shrimp + broccoli + sweet potato mash + brown rice (41 g protein / ~850 cal)

# Days 29–30: Transition Days + Flex Meals

# Purpose

The final two days of your 30-day plan are designed to help you **transition from following a set schedule** to building your own high-protein rhythm.

By now, your fridge and freezer likely hold cooked grains, proteins, soups, and sauces from previous weeks — so instead of starting from scratch, you'll use these as building blocks for fast, satisfying meals.

The goal here is simple:

👉 **Practice flexibility without losing structure.**

You'll combine familiar recipes, leftovers, and quick-prep favorites to build balanced plates that fit your goals.

# Day 29

**Weight Loss Track (~1,650 cal / 120 g protein)**

- Breakfast: Greek yogurt parfait with protein powder + berries (28 g protein / ~350 cal)
- Snack: Boiled eggs (2) + carrots (14 g protein / ~180 cal)
- Lunch: Mix-and-match bowl — ½ cup quinoa + 4 oz chicken + roasted veggies (32 g protein / ~400 cal)
- Snack: Roasted chickpeas or protein ball (12 g protein / ~150 cal)
- Dinner: Shrimp stir-fry leftovers (broccoli, rice, soy sauce, sesame oil) (34 g protein / ~570 cal)

**Muscle Gain Track (~2,350 cal / 156 g protein)**

- Breakfast: Protein smoothie (milk, oats, banana, PB, protein powder) (34 g protein / ~450 cal)
- Snack: Cottage cheese + granola + almonds (20 g protein / ~280 cal)
- Lunch: Build-your-own bowl — 1 cup quinoa + 6 oz chicken + roasted veggies (38 g protein / ~500 cal)
- Snack: Greek yogurt + protein powder + granola (24 g protein / ~300 cal)
- Dinner: Shrimp stir-fry leftovers + added rice or avocado (40 g protein / ~820 cal)

## Day 30

**Weight Loss Track (~1,700 cal / 123 g protein)**

- Breakfast: Protein pancakes + Greek yogurt topping (28 g protein / ~350 cal)
- Snack: Edamame (15 g protein / ~180 cal)
- Lunch: Lentil & veggie soup leftovers (30 g protein / ~400 cal)
- Snack: Cottage cheese + pineapple (13 g protein / ~150 cal)
- Dinner: Garlic butter chicken or salmon leftovers + mixed greens (37 g protein / ~620 cal)

**Muscle Gain Track (~2,400 cal / 159 g protein)**

- Breakfast: Protein pancakes + Greek yogurt + PB drizzle (34 g protein / ~450 cal)
- Snack: Edamame + almonds (20 g protein / ~250 cal)
- Lunch: Lentil & veggie soup + ½ cup rice or 1 slice whole grain bread (38 g protein / ~500 cal)
- Snack: Greek yogurt + protein powder + granola (26 g protein / ~320 cal)
- Dinner: Garlic butter chicken or salmon + mixed greens + brown rice (41 g protein / ~880 cal)

# Tips for Flex Days

- **Use your freezer first.** Rotate any chili, soups, or proteins you froze earlier.
- **Stick to structure, not strictness.** Aim for a protein source, a fiber source, and healthy fat in each meal.
- **Stay hydrated.** Protein metabolism requires water — 80–100 oz per day is ideal.
- **Track what you notice.** You'll now know how your body responds to portions, energy levels, and cravings — write it down.

# Next Steps: Maintaining Momentum

You've built consistency for 30 days — now it's about sustaining it. Use the system you've learned to:

- **Repeat any week** that worked best for your lifestyle.

- **Swap between tracks** as your goals shift (cutting, maintaining, or building).

- **Keep the prep rhythm:** 1 major cook day + 1 mini refresh midweek.

- **Plan, don't improvise:** Even "flex days" work best when intentional.

✓ **Days 29–30 complete your 30-Day High-Protein Meal Plan** — ending with flexibility, autonomy, and mastery over your meal prep rhythm.

# Stacking Note: How to Keep Going After 30 Days

Congratulations — you've just completed a full month of high-protein eating!

Whether your goal was fat loss, muscle gain, or simply consistency, the 30-day plan you followed was designed for adaptability. You've already built the habits, recipes, and prep rhythm that make this lifestyle sustainable long-term.

Now it's time to decide what's next.

## Option 1: Repeat by Goal (Single-Track Stacking)

If your focus is **fat loss**, repeat the **Weight Loss Track** weeks back-to-back for 8–12 weeks.

- Keep portion sizes the same.
- Rotate in new veggies and flavor variations to stay fresh.
- Take one "flex day" each week to practice intuitive balance.

If your goal is **muscle gain,** stack the **Muscle Gain Track** weeks together in the same order.

- Add an extra 100–200 calories per day from carbs or healthy fats if progress slows.
- Use the freezer and Sunday prep structure to stay ahead.
- Track your progress every two weeks — measurements, lifts, or energy levels.

## Option 2: Hybrid Cycling

If you prefer flexibility or want to maintain your results, alternate between tracks.

Example:

- 2 weeks on the **Weight Loss Track** → 2 weeks on the **Muscle Gain Track.** This "protein cycling" approach helps prevent plateaus, supports recovery, and keeps eating enjoyable.

## Option 3: Maintenance Mode

Once you've reached your goal, slide into a **blended approach:**

- Follow the **Muscle Gain Track** portions 3–4 days a week, and

- The **Weight Loss Track** portions 2–3 days a week. This keeps metabolism active, energy steady, and prep simple.

## Your System for Life

By stacking, cycling, or blending these plans, you'll never have to guess what to eat again. You'll understand how to fuel your body, prep confidently, and adjust for any goal — all without starting over.

This isn't a 30-day reset.

It's your **blueprint for high-protein living** — flexible, sustainable, and built to last.

# Chapter 14

# Weekly Meal-Prep Maps

Meal prep isn't just about saving time — it's about creating structure that frees you up to live.

When you know what's in your fridge, you make better choices, waste less food, and hit your protein goals without thinking twice. This chapter gives you simple, repeatable systems that turn one cooking session into **five days of ready-to-eat, high-protein meals.**

Here's what you'll find inside:

- **Cook Once, Eat Five Days:** Step-by-step prep maps that show exactly how to batch-cook proteins, grains, and vegetables so you can assemble fresh combinations all week long.

- **Storage & Reheating Chart:** A quick-reference guide for how long each food keeps, whether it can be frozen, and how to reheat it safely without drying it out or losing nutrients.

- **Choose Your Batch Base:** A mix-and-match system that lets you pick one protein, one starch, and one veggie to form your week's foundation — with seasoning ideas and flavor variations for every combo.

Think of this chapter as your **kitchen GPS.** You'll get a visual map for turning a Sunday cooking session into grab-and-go breakfasts, lunches, and dinners that fit your plan — no burnout, no boring repeats, no wasted effort.

By the end, you'll know how to design a full week of meals in under two hours — and finally make "meal prep" a habit that works for real life.

# Cook Once, Eat 5 Days

*Batch once, eat better all week.*

Meal prep doesn't have to mean eating the same bowl five days in a row.

By cooking one versatile protein, starch, and vegetable base, you can mix, season, and combine them into new flavors every day — without extra cooking or burnout.

Here are a few ready-to-follow examples to get you started.

## Map 1: Chicken + Quinoa + Broccoli

**Batch Cook:**

- 2 lbs chicken breast (grilled or baked)
- 3 cups cooked quinoa
- 4 cups steamed broccoli

**Use It 5 Ways:**

| Day | Meal | Flavor Remix | Notes |
|---|---|---|---|
| Mon | Chicken & Broccoli Bowl | Add soy sauce + sesame oil + green onions | Asian-inspired power bowl |
| Tue | Chicken Quinoa Salad | Toss with spinach, lemon juice, olive oil | Light & refreshing lunch |
| Wed | Chicken "Fried Rice" | Sauté all bases with egg + low-sodium soy | Quick skillet meal |
| Thu | Chicken Tacos | Wrap in whole-wheat tortillas + salsa | High-protein, fiber-rich |
| | | | |

| | | | |
|---|---|---|---|
| **Fri** | Chicken & Broccoli Casserole | Bake with low-fat cheese + yogurt sauce | Comfort food done clean |

**Batch Time:** 90 minutes →

**Meals Ready:** 5

**Protein per Day:** ~32–38 g

**Map 2: Ground Turkey + Brown Rice + Peppers & Onions**

**Batch Cook:**

- 2 lbs lean ground turkey

- 3 cups cooked brown rice

- 3 cups sautéed bell peppers and onions

**Use It 5 Ways:**

| Day | Meal | Flavor Remix | Notes |
|---|---|---|---|
| **Mon** | Turkey Burrito Bowl | Add black beans, salsa, and avocado | Southwest-style bowl |
| **Tue** | Turkey Lettuce Wraps | Add shredded carrots, soy-ginger sauce | Fresh, low-carb |
| **Wed** | Turkey Fried Rice | Stir-fry all bases with egg | Reheat-friendly |
| **Thu** | Turkey & Rice Stuffed Peppers | Bake with tomato sauce + mozzarella | Great freezer meal |
| **Fri** | Turkey Breakfast Scramble | Add eggs + spinach | Fast high-protein start |

**Batch Time:** 1 hour →

**Meals Ready:** 5

**Protein per Day:** ~30–36 g

**Map 3: Salmon + Sweet Potato + Asparagus**

**Batch Cook:**

- 4 salmon fillets (6 oz each, baked or air-fried)

- 3 medium sweet potatoes (roasted or mashed)

- 1 bunch asparagus (steamed or roasted)

**Use It 5 Ways:**

| Day | Meal | Flavor Remix | Notes |
|---|---|---|---|
| **Mon** | Salmon Power Bowl | Add quinoa + tahini dressing | Heart-healthy start |
| **Tue** | Salmon Tacos | Shred salmon + cabbage slaw + lime | Easy 10-min meal |
| **Wed** | Salmon Salad | Toss with spinach + lemon yogurt sauce | Light lunch |
| **Thu** | Salmon Cakes | Mix leftovers with egg + breadcrumbs | Crispy and portable |
| **Fri** | Sweet Potato Mash Bowl | Add asparagus + yogurt drizzle | Comfort meal for the week's end |

**Batch Time:** 75 minutes →

**Meals Ready:** 5

**Protein per Day:** ~32–40 g

**Map 4: Tofu + Jasmine Rice + Mixed Veggies (Vegan)**

**Batch Cook:**

- 1 block extra-firm tofu (baked or pan-seared)

- 3 cups cooked jasmine rice

- 3 cups mixed vegetables (broccoli, peppers, edamame)

**Use It 5 Ways:**

| Day | Meal | Flavor Remix | Notes |
|---|---|---|---|
| **Mon** | Tofu Stir-Fry | Add teriyaki sauce + sesame seeds | Classic vegan prep |
| **Tue** | Curry Tofu Bowl | Simmer with coconut milk + curry paste | Rich & warming |
| **Wed** | Tofu Burrito Bowl | Add salsa + avocado + black beans | High-fiber lunch |
| **Thu** | Crispy Tofu Wrap | Add hummus + spinach + carrot ribbons | Great cold lunch |
| **Fri** | Tofu Fried Rice | Add egg or Just Egg + soy sauce | Quick 10-min dinner |

**Batch Time:** 1 hour →

**Meals Ready:** 5

**Protein per Day:** ~26–34 g

**Map 5: Beef + Quinoa + Zucchini & Spinach**

**Batch Cook:**

- 1½ lbs lean ground beef

- 3 cups cooked quinoa

- 3 cups sautéed zucchini and spinach

**Use It 5 Ways:**

| Day | Meal | Flavor Remix | Notes |
|---|---|---|---|
| **Mon** | Beef Power Bowl | Add chili flakes + tomato sauce | Bold & savory |
| **Tue** | Beef & Quinoa Stuffed Peppers | Bake with mozzarella | Meal-prep favorite |
| **Wed** | Beef Tacos | Add salsa + shredded lettuce | Fast high-protein dinner |
| **Thu** | Beef Breakfast Bowl | Add scrambled eggs + spinach | Morning protein boost |
| **Fri** | Beef Chili | Add black beans + diced tomatoes | One-pot freezer win |

**Batch Time:** 90 minutes →

**Meals Ready:** 5

**Protein per Day:** ~33–40 g

✓ These **"Cook Once, Eat 5 Days"** maps are flexible templates.

You can substitute any protein (like shrimp or tempeh), grain (like rice, quinoa, or farro), or vegetable (fresh, frozen, or roasted) — the structure stays the same.

# Storage & Reheating Chart

*How long your meal-prep staples stay fresh — and how to bring them back to life.*

| Food | Fridge Life ❄ | Freezer Life ❄ | Reheat Method 🔥 | Tips for Best Results |
|------|---------------|----------------|------------------|-----------------------|
| **Chicken (cooked)** | 4 days | 2 months | Microwave 1–2 min or skillet 5 min | Add a splash of broth to keep it moist |
| **Ground turkey/beef** | 4 days | 2 months | Skillet 5–7 min | Reheat covered to prevent drying |
| **Fish (salmon, cod, tilapia)** | 3 days | 2 months | Bake or skillet 6–8 min | Avoid microwave to prevent overcooking |
| **Shrimp** | 3 days | 1 month | Sauté 3–5 min | Reheat gently — shrimp dries quickly |
| **Tofu (cooked/baked)** | 5 days | 2 months | Skillet or air fryer 5 min | Add soy or teriyaki for moisture |
| **Quinoa / Rice (cooked)** | 5 days | 3 months | Microwave 1 min or steam 3 min | Add 1 tsp water before reheating |
| **Sweet potatoes (roasted/mashed)** | 5 days | 3 months | Microwave 1–2 min | Great for mash or grain bowls |
| | | | Microwave | Reheat only |

| | | | | |
|---|---|---|---|---|
| **Vegetables (steamed/roasted)** | 4–5 days | 2 months | 1 min or skillet 3–5 min | once to preserve texture |
| **Soups & stews** | 5 days | 3 months | Microwave or simmer 5–8 min | Freeze in single-serve containers |
| **Eggs (hard-boiled)** | 7 days | Do not freeze | Eat cold or slice into meals | Store unpeeled for longer freshness |
| **Protein pancakes/waffles** | 5 days | 2 months | Microwave for 30 sec or toaster | Freeze in layers with parchment |
| **Protein balls/bars** | 7 days | 3 months | No reheating | Store in an airtight container |
| **Greek yogurt/cottage cheese** | 7 days | Do not freeze | Eat cold | Great protein snack base |
| **Chili or lentil soup** | 5–6 days | 3 months | Microwave or simmer 5 min | Thaw overnight before reheating |

# Quick Storage Tips

- ❄ **Freeze in portions:** Divide meals into single servings before freezing.

- 🗓 **Label and date everything:** Use masking tape or freezer labels — 30 days pass faster than you think.

- 🔥 **Reheat once:** Reheating multiple times can reduce quality and increase food safety risk.

- ⬦ **Add moisture back:** When reheating meats or grains, add 1–2 tsp water, broth, or olive oil to revive texture.

# Choose Your Batch Base

*One protein. One starch. One vegetable. Endless combinations.*

Batch cooking works best when it's flexible. Instead of memorizing recipes, think in **building blocks:**

- **Protein** fuels recovery and satiety.

- **Starch** provides energy and fiber.

- **Vegetables** add volume, nutrients, and flavor.

Mix and match from the chart below to **create your own meal-prep map** — then use spices and sauces to keep things exciting week after week.

## Protein Bases

*(Cook 2–4 lbs once for the week)*

| Protein | Cook Method | Flavor Ideas | Pairs Best With |
|---|---|---|---|
| Chicken breast | Grill, bake, or slow cook | Lemon herb • BBQ • Teriyaki • Garlic butter | Rice, quinoa, sweet potatoes |
| Ground turkey | Sauté or bake | Taco spice • Italian herb • Curry • Soy-ginger | Brown rice, pasta, wraps |
| Salmon | Bake or air-fry | Lemon dill • Honey mustard • Cajun • Garlic butter | Quinoa, roasted potatoes |
| Shrimp | Sauté or grill | Chili-lime • Garlic butter • Teriyaki • Paprika-lemon | Rice, noodles, zoodles |
| Tofu (extra-firm) | Bake or pan-sear | Teriyaki • Peanut • Curry • Smoked paprika | Jasmine rice, quinoa |

| | | | |
|---|---|---|---|
| Ground beef (lean) | Sauté | Taco • Chili • Garlic herb • Mediterranean | Rice, couscous, wraps |
| Lentils / beans | Simmer | Cumin • Curry • Tomato-herb • Lemon-garlic | Quinoa, farro, brown rice |
| Eggs | Boil, scramble, or bake | Plain • Salsa • Pesto • Veggie-loaded | Potatoes, toast, wraps |

## Starch Bases

*(Cook 3–4 cups for the week)*

| Starch | Cook Method | Flavor Ideas | Storage Tip |
|---|---|---|---|
| Quinoa | Boil | Garlic + lemon • Cilantro-lime | Add 1 tsp olive oil before chilling |
| Brown rice | Steam or boil | Soy-ginger • Cajun • Herb butter | Store with 1 tbsp water to keep soft |
| Sweet potatoes | Roast or mash | Cinnamon • Chili-lime • Rosemary | Store in airtight container |
| White potatoes | Boil or roast | Garlic-parsley • Paprika • Olive oil | Mash for bowls or breakfast |
| Pasta (whole grain) | Boil | Italian herb • Pesto • Lemon garlic | Toss with olive oil to prevent sticking |
| Couscous or farro | Boil | Curry • Tomato-basil • Za'atar | Freeze well for quick meals |
| Oats | Overnight or cook | Cinnamon • Vanilla • PB-chocolate | Perfect for breakfasts/snacks |

## Vegetable Bases

*(Prep 4–6 cups mixed veggies for the week)*

| Veggie | Cook Method | Flavor Ideas | Pro Tip |
|---|---|---|---|
| Broccoli | Steam or roast | Garlic butter • Lemon zest | Slightly undercook for reheating |
| Zucchini | Sauté or roast | Italian herb • Soy-ginger | Great for stir-fries or bowls |
| Bell peppers | Roast or sauté | Fajita-style • Mediterranean | Sweeten as they roast |
| Spinach / kale | Steam or sauté | Olive oil + garlic | Freeze extra into smoothie cubes |
| Carrots | Roast or steam | Honey-glaze • Cumin • Thyme | Slice for snacks or side dishes |
| Asparagus | Roast or steam | Lemon-parmesan • Garlic | Store upright in water if fresh |
| Green beans | Steam or sauté | Garlic • Soy • Lemon pepper | Best eaten within 3–4 days |
| Mixed veggies (frozen) | Steam | Curry • Cajun • Sesame | Instant backup for any meal |

# Build Your Own Batch Map

*Pick 1 protein + 1 starch + 1 veggie, then flavor it your way:*

| Base Combo | Flavor Theme | Sauce or Topping |
|---|---|---|
| Chicken + quinoa + broccoli | Asian | Teriyaki + sesame seeds |
| Salmon + sweet potato + asparagus | Mediterranean | Olive oil + lemon + dill |
| Tofu + brown rice + mixed veggies | Thai | Peanut sauce + chili flakes |
| Ground turkey + pasta + spinach | Italian | Marinara + Parmesan |
| Lentils + couscous + carrots | Middle Eastern | Tahini + lemon juice |
| Shrimp + rice + zucchini | Cajun | Garlic butter + parsley |
| Beef + quinoa + peppers | Tex-Mex | Salsa + avocado |

# Batch Builder Formula

For easy portioning:

- **Protein**: 4–6 oz (weight loss) or 6–8 oz (muscle gain)
- **Starch**: ½ cup cooked (weight loss) or 1 cup cooked (muscle gain)
- **Veggies**: 1–2 cups any mix
- **Flavor**: 1–2 tsp sauce or spice blend

Total prep time: **90 minutes or less** for a full week of mix-and-match meals.

# Chapter 15

# Smart Indexes & Quick Tools

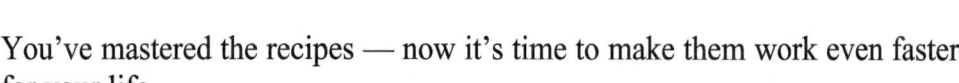

You've mastered the recipes — now it's time to make them work even faster for your life.

This chapter turns the entire cookbook into a **customizable system** you can search, sort, and use on the fly. Whether you're counting protein grams, short on time, or cooking on a budget, these quick tools help you find exactly what you need in seconds.

Here's what's inside:

- **Recipe Index by Protein Power:** Organized by 20g, 30g, and 40g+ per serving so you can match meals to your daily target.

- **Quick-Find Index:** Search recipes by cook time, appliance (air fryer, Instant Pot, sheet pan, slow cooker), or price point — perfect for busy weeks.

- **"Tonight I Need..." Flowchart:** A simple visual guide to help you choose the right recipe when time or energy is low — from 15-minute fixes to full batch-cook sessions.

Think of this as your **navigation dashboard** for the whole book — a way to plan smarter, save time, and always have a high-protein meal ready for whatever life throws your way.

# Smart Recipe Index

## By Protein Power (grams per serving)

**20g Range** — Light meals & snacks

- Greek Yogurt Parfait
- Edamame with Sea Salt
- Cottage Cheese & Fruit Cups
- Protein Balls
- Tofu Stir-Fry
- Protein Smoothies (base recipes)

**30g Range** — Balanced everyday meals

- Lentil & Quinoa Buddha Bowl
- Turkey & Avocado Lettuce Wraps
- Tuna & White Bean Salad
- Chicken Quinoa Salad
- Greek Chickpea Power Salad
- Garlic Butter Shrimp Stir-Fry
- Salmon Power Bowl
- Tofu Curry Bowl
- Ground Turkey Burrito Bowl

**40g+ Range** — High-performance & post-workout meals

- Sheet-Pan Lemon Herb Salmon with Veggies

- Garlic Butter Chicken & Broccoli Skillet
- Beef & Lentil Chili
- Shrimp Fried "Rice" (Cauliflower Base)
- One-Pot Turkey & Lentil Chili
- Baked Cod with Sweet Potato Mash
- Chicken & Lentil Stew
- Turkey Meatballs with Whole Wheat Pasta

# By Cook Time

### 15 Minutes or Less

- Protein Smoothies
- Cottage Cheese Bowls
- Tuna & Avocado Cucumber Roll-Ups
- Scrambled Eggs with Spinach
- Greek Yogurt Ranch Dip
- Edamame Snacks

### 30 Minutes or Less

- Garlic Butter Shrimp Stir-Fry
- Chicken & Quinoa Salad
- Turkey Lettuce Wraps
- Tofu Stir-Fry
- Salmon Power Bowl
- Turkey Breakfast Scramble
- Protein Pancakes or Mug Cake

**Batch or Make-Ahead (45–90 Minutes)**

- Lentil & Quinoa Buddha Bowl
- Beef & Lentil Chili
- Sheet-Pan Chicken & Veggies
- Turkey & Rice Stuffed Peppers
- Chicken & Broccoli Casserole
- Big-Batch Turkey Meatballs
- Slow Cooker Pulled BBQ Turkey
- Lentil Soup or Stew

**Freezer-Friendly Meals**

- Turkey Chili
- Lentil Soup
- Chicken & Veggie Sheet-Pan Meals
- Protein Pancakes
- Sweet Potato Mash Bowls
- Baked Salmon Portions

# By Appliance

**Air Fryer**

- Lemon Herb Salmon Fillets
- Crispy Tofu Bites
- Chicken & Veggie Sheet-Pan Meals
- Protein Pancakes (reheat option)

**Instant Pot / Pressure Cooker**

- Lentil & Turkey Soup
- Beef & Lentil Chili
- Chicken & Quinoa Bowl Base
- Turkey & Veggie Curry

## Slow Cooker

- Pulled BBQ Turkey
- Chicken & Veggie Stew
- Lentil Soup with Sweet Potato
- Turkey Chili

## Oven / Sheet Pan

- Sheet-Pan Chicken & Veggies
- Garlic Butter Salmon
- Turkey Stuffed Peppers
- Baked Cod with Mashed Potatoes
- Chicken & Broccoli Casserole

## Skillet / Stovetop

- Garlic Butter Chicken & Broccoli Skillet
- Shrimp Stir-Fry
- Turkey Breakfast Scramble
- Quinoa "Fried Rice"
- Tofu Veggie Stir-Fry

# By Budget Level

## § Budget-Friendly

- Tuna & White Bean Salad
- Lentil & Quinoa Buddha Bowl
- Egg Scramble with Spinach
- Turkey Chili
- Edamame Snack Cups
- Chicken & Veggie Sheet-Pan Meal

## §§ Mid-Range

- Shrimp Stir-Fry
- Baked Cod with Sweet Potato Mash
- Chicken & Lentil Stew
- Greek Chickpea Power Salad
- Turkey & Quinoa Stuffed Peppers

## §§§ Premium Protein Meals

- Lemon Herb Salmon Power Bowl
- Garlic Butter Shrimp Stir-Fry
- Beef & Lentil Chili
- Salmon Cakes

Chicken & Broccoli Casserole (high-protein version with Greek yogurt)

# "Tonight, I Need..." Flowchart

*Your quick-decision guide to picking the perfect high-protein meal — even when you're tired, busy, or low on groceries.*

## Step 1 — How much time do you have?

⏱ **15 minutes or less** → Go to **Quick Fix Zone**

⏱ **30 minutes** → Go to **Everyday Dinners**

⏱ **45–90 minutes (or Sunday prep)** → Go to **Batch & Freeze Zone**

## Quick Fix Zone (15 min or less)

Perfect for busy nights, post-workouts, or *"I can't even"* evenings.

Choose your path:

🔦 **Need something cold?** → Greek Yogurt Parfait • Cottage Cheese & Fruit Cups • Protein Smoothie

🔥 **Need something hot?** → Scrambled Eggs with Spinach • Tuna & Avocado Wraps • Edamame Snack Bowl

💡 *Tip:* Double your serving and you've got tomorrow's snack ready too.

## Everyday Dinners (30 min)

*Fast, fresh, balanced — ideal for weeknights.*

## Choose your craving:

🍱 **Light & fresh** → Chicken & Quinoa Salad • Shrimp Stir-Fry • Tofu Veggie Bowl

🍲 **Comforting & savory** → Turkey Lettuce Wraps • Garlic Butter Chicken Skillet • Salmon Power Bowl

🥣 **Budget-friendly** → Lentil & Quinoa Buddha Bowl • Tuna & White

Bean Salad

💡 *Tip:* Pick two recipes, cook once, and alternate leftovers for variety.

# Batch & Freeze Zone (45–90 min)

*Perfect for Sundays or slow evenings when you want to stock up.*

# Choose your strategy:

🍲 **Slow Cooker / Instant Pot** → Turkey Chili • Chicken & Lentil Stew • Lentil Soup with Sweet Potato

🔥 **Oven / Sheet Pan** → Sheet-Pan Chicken & Veggies • Baked Cod with Mashed Potatoes • Turkey Stuffed Peppers

🥫 **Freezer-friendly bulk** → Big-Batch Turkey Meatballs • Beef & Lentil Chili • Protein Pancakes

💡 *Tip:* Label with the date and protein per serving — future you will thank you.

# Step 2 — What tool do you want to use tonight?

- 🔥 **Skillet / Stovetop:** Garlic Butter Chicken, Shrimp Fried "Rice," Tofu Stir-Fry

- 🍽 **Oven / Air Fryer:** Lemon Herb Salmon, Sheet-Pan Chicken, Turkey Stuffed Peppers

- 🕐 **Slow Cooker / Instant Pot:** Pulled BBQ Turkey, Lentil Soup, Chicken Curry

💡 *Tip:* All recipes list cook times and macros — just match what you have to your goal.

# Step 3 — What's your energy level?

😵 **Running on fumes?** → Smoothies, Wraps, or Scrambles

💪 **Have some motivation?** → Stir-fries, Skillets, or Salads

🔥 **Feeling productive?** → Batch-cook chili or casseroles

**Step 4 — Choose your win**

✔ **Need fast fuel?** → Quick Fix Zone

✔ **Need comfort food?** → Everyday Dinners

✔ **Need to get ahead?** → Batch & Freeze Zone

☑ Keep this flowchart bookmarked or taped to your fridge.

It turns the entire cookbook into a **choose-your-own-adventure for healthy, high-protein living** — no guesswork, no stress, just smart choices that fit your time, mood, and goals.

# Conclusion

# **Your Protein-Powered Life**

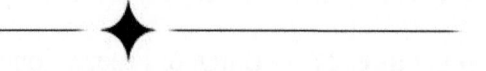

You've done more than follow recipes — you've built a system that works for your real life.

You've learned how to cook smarter, not longer. You've seen how the right balance of protein, prep, and planning can simplify your days, fuel your energy, and move you closer to your goals — one meal at a time.

Along the way, you discovered that "high-protein" isn't a dict — it's a foundation. It's a way to eat that keeps you strong, steady, and satisfied, whether you're chasing fitness goals, staying active as you age, or just trying to eat better without overthinking it.

By now, your kitchen is more than a workspace — it's your launchpad. You've mastered batch cooking, built confidence in your prep rhythm, and created go-to meals that fit your taste, budget, and schedule. You've learned that eating well doesn't have to be complicated. It just has to be consistent.

As you move forward, keep using the tools from this book:

- Your **meal-prep maps** to save time and reduce stress.
- Your **batch-based system** to customize your meals.
- Your **flowcharts and indexes** to make fast, smart choices.

Every meal you prep is a small investment in a stronger you — one that pays back in energy, focus, and freedom.

So celebrate your progress, trust your process, and keep going.

Your high-protein lifestyle isn't something you have to maintain — it's something you now *live*.

You've got the recipes, the roadmap, and the rhythm.

Now it's your turn to make it your own.

# Thank You for Cooking with Me

If you've made it this far, you've done something most people never do — you've taken real, sustainable action toward better eating and better living.

By now, you've seen how simple it can be to stay consistent when your meals work *for* you instead of against you. My hope is that this book has helped you feel more confident in your kitchen, more relaxed in your routine, and more connected to your health goals — one meal at a time.

If this cookbook made your meal prep easier, your food tastier, or your days smoother, I'd love to hear from you. Your feedback doesn't just help me — it helps other readers discover tools that make healthy living feel doable, too.

💬 **Would you take a quick moment to leave a review on Amazon?**

It only takes a minute, but it makes a world of difference.

Your review helps this book reach more people who are ready to eat better, live stronger, and simplify their health journey — just like you.

Thank you again for inviting me into your kitchen.

Here's to your next batch, your next goal, and your next great meal.

Keep cooking. Keep going.

And remember — progress is built one prep day at a time.

# Appendix
# Resources & Conversions

## Protein Cheat Sheet

*A quick guide to everyday foods and their approximate protein per serving.*

| Food | Serving Size | Protein (g) |
|---|---|---|
| Chicken breast (cooked) | 4 oz | 35 g |
| Ground turkey (93% lean) | 4 oz | 30 g |
| Salmon or cod (cooked) | 4 oz | 25 g |
| Shrimp | 4 oz | 22 g |
| Lean ground beef | 4 oz | 28 g |
| Eggs | 2 large | 12 g |
| Egg whites | 4 | 14 g |
| Greek yogurt (plain, nonfat) | ¾ cup | 17 g |
| Cottage cheese (low-fat) | ½ cup | 14 g |
| Tofu (extra firm) | 4 oz | 10 g |
| Tempeh | 4 oz | 20 g |
| Lentils (cooked) | 1 cup | 18 g |
| Black beans | 1 cup | 15 g |
| Edamame | 1 cup | 17 g |
| Protein powder (whey or plant) | 1 scoop | 20–25 g |

💡 *Tip*: Pair plant proteins like lentils, beans, and quinoa for a complete amino acid profile.

## Quick Kitchen Conversions

| Measurement | Equivalent |
|---|---|
| 1 tablespoon (Tbsp) | 3 teaspoons (tsp) |
| 1 cup | 8 fluid ounces (fl oz) |
| 1 pint | 2 cups |
| 1 quart | 4 cups |
| 1 pound (lb) | 16 ounces (oz) |
| 1 ounce | 28 grams |
| 100 grams | 3.5 ounces |
| 1 tablespoon oil/nut butter | ~120 calories |
| 1 scoop protein powder | ~30 grams (varies by brand) |

💡 *Tip*: Keep a small digital scale handy for more consistent tracking of protein and calories.

# Macro Balance Reference

*How to estimate balanced meal ratios for different goals.*

| Goal | Protein | Carbs | Fats | Example Meal |
|---|---|---|---|---|
| Fat Loss | 40% | 30% | 30% | Chicken + broccoli + quinoa |
| Maintenance | 35% | 35% | 30% | Shrimp stir-fry + rice + veggies |
| Muscle Gain | 30% | 45% | 25% | Turkey chili + rice + avocado |
| Active Aging | 35% | 40% | 25% | Salmon + sweet potato + spinach |

💡 *Tip*: Adjust carbs up or down by 10% based on activity level — protein stays steady.

# Pantry Refill Checklist

*Keep these staples on hand for easy high-protein meal prep.*

## Proteins:

- Chicken breast, ground turkey, eggs, Greek yogurt, cottage cheese
- Tofu, tempeh, lentils, beans, canned tuna or salmon, protein powder

## Carbs & Grains:

- Quinoa, brown rice, oats, sweet potatoes, whole wheat pasta, couscous

## Healthy Fats:

- Olive oil, avocado, nut butter, almonds, chia seeds, flaxseed

## Veggies & Flavor:

- Broccoli, spinach, peppers, onions, carrots, mixed greens
- Garlic, lemon, herbs, low-sodium soy sauce, salsa, mustard, yogurt-based sauces

## Storage Supplies:

- Meal-prep containers (glass or BPA-free)
- Freezer bags & labels
- Mini jars for sauces & dressings

## Helpful Kitchen Tools

- 🍳 Nonstick skillet or cast-iron pan
- 🍲 Slow cooker or Instant Pot
- 🍱 Air fryer or sheet pan set
- ⚖️ Food scale
- 🥣 Mixing bowls with lids
- 🧊 Ice cube trays (for freezing sauces or broths)

💡 *Tip:* Choose durable, stackable containers to make your weekly prep flow smoother and save fridge space.